AF588038

Health Informatics

This series is directed to healthcare professionals leading the transformation of healthcare by using information and knowledge. For over 20 years, Health Informatics has offered a broad range of titles: some address specific professions such as nursing, medicine, and health administration; others cover special areas of practice such as trauma and radiology; still other books in the series focus on interdisciplinary issues, such as the computer based patient record, electronic health records, and networked healthcare systems. Editors and authors, eminent experts in their fields, offer their accounts of innovations in health informatics. Increasingly, these accounts go beyond hardware and software to address the role of information in influencing the transformation of healthcare delivery systems around the world. The series also increasingly focuses on the users of the information and systems: the organizational, behavioral, and societal changes that accompany the diffusion of information technology in health services environments.

Developments in healthcare delivery are constant; in recent years, bioinformatics has emerged as a new field in health informatics to support emerging and ongoing developments in molecular biology. At the same time, further evolution of the field of health informatics is reflected in the introduction of concepts at the macro or health systems delivery level with major national initiatives related to electronic health records (EHR), data standards, and public health informatics.

These changes will continue to shape health services in the twenty-first century. By making full and creative use of the technology to tame data and to transform information, Health Informatics will foster the development and use of new knowledge in healthcare.

Ursula H. Hübner • Giovanni Rubeis
Connie White Delaney • Marion J. Ball
Editors

Bridging Artificial and Human Intelligence

Implementation Strategies and Case Studies in Healthcare

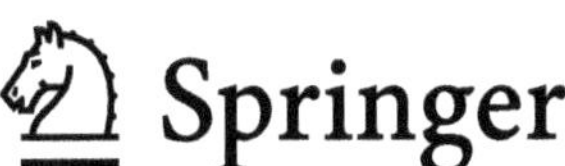

Editors
Ursula H. Hübner
School of Business Management
and Social Sciences
Osnabrück University Applied Sciences
Osnabrück, Germany

Giovanni Rubeis
Institut for Ethics and History of Medicine
University of Greifswald
Greifswald, Germany

Connie White Delaney
School of Nursing
University of Minnesota
Minneapolis, MN, USA

Marion J. Ball
Center for Innovation in Health
Informatics (CIHI)
The University of Texas at Arlington
Arlington, TX, USA

ISSN 1431-1917 ISSN 2197-3741 (electronic)
Health Informatics
ISBN 978-3-032-11937-7 ISBN 978-3-032-11938-4 (eBook)
https://doi.org/10.1007/978-3-032-11938-4

This Springer imprint is published by the registered company Springer Nature Switzerland AG
The registered company address is: Gewerbestrasse 11, 6330 Cham, Switzerland

I dedicate this book to my husband whose humor and wit is a constant source of mental refreshment.

Ursula H. Hübner

To the memory of my father who taught me the most important lesson of all.

Giovanni Rubeis

This book is dedicated to all people and care organizations for their insights and requests that drive informatics innovation.

Connie White Delaney

This book is dedicated to Raj and Indra Nooyi, whose generosity and vision have advanced the integration of engineering and healthcare informatics, strengthening scholarship and education for future generations.

Marion J. Ball

Foreword

This ambitious text covers a broad spectrum of topics related to the introduction of artificial intelligence (AI) into healthcare broadly. The focus is on health informatics, how it could change, how it needs to change, and how we must think about those changes as it relates to this new technology. As an internist whose subspecialty and primary focus has been on health informatics, I look back on my 60+ years of trying to make some of those changes and, after reading this book, only wish I could do it all again in this exciting new era.

To introduce these topics, I will focus on just one of the areas this text will cover. Although there are many areas of healthcare informatics that have demonstrated remarkable achievements, for better or worse and whether we like it or not, it is the history of electronic health records (EHRs) that has most characterized our health informatics subspecialty. That history is about to change (for the better) with AI.

I have lived and worked through the entire history of EHRs. I learned Fortran in college in the 1950s, more advanced software in medical school in the 1960s, and developed my first crude EHR in the late 1960s at Johns Hopkins. Developing multiple EHRs subsequently, including two commercial products still in use today, I have personally experienced this entire history. That history is mixed.

The motivation of us early EHR pioneers was to replace the paper chart which had three major flaws: (1) it could only be in one place at a time and often not where it was needed, (2) it was frequently illegible and poorly organized, and (3) it was fragmented into multiple paper components if the patient was seen by multiple organizations.

By and large, the early EHRs of the 1970s and 1980s solved the first two of those paper chart problems. They did not solve the fragmentation problem, nor have we yet done so. Although HL7 and other communication standards, as well as local and wide area networking technologies, proliferated in the 1980s and 1990s, true open architecture in healthcare did not succeed commercially, and we continue to have fragmented electronic health records.

Nonetheless, we EHR developers focused our attention on an entirely new use of the medical record, one not even contemplated during the paper chart phase: decision support. It was obvious from the beginning that the computer could be used for more than display and communication of patient information; specifically, it could also be used to reduce clinical errors of omission and commission. To do this, however, it required that the data entered into the EHR be coded in a manner that would allow the software to automate error checking. Free text could not be coded. Since the typical input mode up to the 1980s was either verbal dictation and transcription, typing text, or handwriting, the notion of "structured text" had to be introduced into all EHRs. Although this enabled the massive proliferation of decision support software into all EHRs since the 1980s, this turned out to be a mixed blessing at best.

Simultaneous with the entry of structured text was the realization by healthcare financial administrators that this same coding ability could enable the EHR to be the source of billing information. When the American Medical Association, which owns the CPT coding system used by health insurers for billing, agreed to develop a new system for billing for patient encounters that was based on the clinicians' encounter note entry (E&M codes), the structured text technology of EHRs became usurped for billing purposes. That basically doomed the EHR as a welcome tool for clinicians.

We are all familiar with the resulting dissatisfaction of clinicians using EHRs: endless clicking on input lists to enter history and physical findings, voluminous encounter notes spitting back those lists on display, clinician burn-out from the hours spent at a computer screen, and distrust of the accuracy of the patient data resulting from attempts to ease the input through defaults, "pull forward," and other gimmicks to produce an encounter note. Decision support alert fatigue compounds all these other issues. Although few wish to return to the paper record, it would be difficult for those of us who have labored in this field to declare that our characterizing contribution—the EHR—is a huge success.

So why am I optimistic regarding the future of this one sentinel aspect of health informatics—the EHR? AI makes structured text obsolete. The EHR of the future, including new ones being introduced today, will solve the biggest single impediment to user-friendly EHRs: Endless clicking. Clinicians will once again be able to do what they always felt comfortable doing. Talking. They will just verbalize the history, physical exam, and any other component of a SOAP note they wish to document. No more scribes to try to ease the input burden. I think back to the 1990s when voice recognition technology was being introduced. I remarked then that my only hope was that voice recognition technology would fail. It would revert us back to free text encounter notes without any ability to do decision support. The difference with AI rather than transcriptionists is that LLMs "understand" natural language. Coding of free text is now possible.

More importantly, decision support will finally exit the cumbersome and costly "rules" era. No longer will software developers need to code and maintain endless guidelines, templates, and customized rules for every aspect of clinical knowledge. I envision the future input of SOAP notes to consist of the Subjective and Objective components being verbalized as described above and the Assessment and Plan components presented to the clinician by the AI for review and editing. The difference from what decision support has always required in the past is that this "generative" component of the AI system will utilize not only information just verbalized by the clinician but also any information about the patient *and* about clinical knowledge accessible electronically. Its "intelligence" will not be dependent on pre-programmed rules but rather AI-determined knowledge available anywhere on the Internet continually evolving as that knowledge evolves.

All of this will not happen instantaneously and without problems. We will still need health informaticians to make this happen safely. We will still need research and testing to detect and resolve errors (or "hallucinations"). We will still need regulations and a revised approval process for the EHRs. We will still need to solve our interoperability problem to allow the AI access to the most complete data. We will need to rethink and redefine the relevance and concepts of terminologies, coding systems and standards. And, most importantly, we will need to dramatically upgrade our clinician education programs to optimize the use of this exciting new technology.

I have focused on this one example of many that will be discussed in this text. Similar revolutions of thinking are taking place in each one of them. Enjoy the journey!

IKnowMed
Berkeley, CA, USA

Donald W. Simborg

Foreword

As we embark on a journey that intertwines the realms of human intellect and artificial intelligence (AI), the book *Bridging Artificial and Human Intelligence: Implementation Strategies and Case Studies in Healthcare* serves as a guiding light. It illuminates the path toward a future where AI and human intelligence not only coexist but collaborate in the realm of healthcare, fostering a synergy that could revolutionize the industry.

This work, by Ursula H. Hübner, Giovanni Rubeis, Connie W. Delaney, and Marion J. Ball, is not just a book—it's a revelation. It portrays a future where AI is not seen as a threat but as a valuable partner to human intelligence. The authors, with their rich experience and knowledge in healthcare informatics, AI, and leadership, are researchers and practitioners from various fields, across academia and industry. They reflect diverse geographic regions and share their unique insights and perspectives to bear on the complex and rapidly evolving landscape of AI in healthcare. The editors have created a comprehensive guide that navigates the complex landscape of AI in healthcare, providing a roadmap for those who dare to venture into this exciting territory. Their collective wisdom, distilled into the pages of this book, provides a roadmap for navigating this challenging terrain.

Bridging Artificial and Human Intelligence: Implementation Strategies and Case Studies in Healthcare offers a thorough exploration of how AI can be strategically implemented in the healthcare sector. It discusses how AI can improve efficiency, enhance patient outcomes, and foster a deeper understanding of complex medical phenomena.

The book's intended audience is broad and diverse. It caters to clinicians, professionals, and decision-makers seeking to understand both the benefits and limitations of AI in tandem with human involvement. It also serves as a valuable resource for graduate students seeking to enhance their understanding of AI's role in healthcare.

The book offers guidance on how to execute strategies, as well as the ethical and legal standards pertinent to AI integration. It surpasses theory, presenting a range of captivating case studies that reveal a distinctive view on the mutual relationship between human decision-making and AI. These case studies show how they can coexist and cooperate to transform healthcare.

The impact of this symbiosis on healthcare providers, patients, and families is profound. For healthcare providers, the integration of AI can lead to more accurate diagnoses, personalized treatment plans, and improved patient monitoring. It can also reduce the workload, allowing them to focus more on patient care rather than administrative tasks.

For patients, AI can provide a more personalized healthcare experience. It can help in predicting health risks, managing chronic conditions, and even in recovery processes. AI can provide patients with access to healthcare services from the comfort of their homes, making healthcare more accessible. For families, AI can help them stay informed about the health of their loved ones and assist in managing their health. AI can also provide support in making informed decisions about the healthcare of their family members.

I am profoundly grateful for my professional relationships with the authors of this transformative book. Their expertise and dedication have been instrumental in shaping this book and the future of healthcare. Their work is a testament to the power of collaboration and the potential of AI in healthcare.

As you turn the pages of this book, you will be inspired and enlightened by the possibilities that lie ahead. I hope you will see, as I do, a future where AI and human intelligence work collectively to provide better healthcare for all. A future where AI is not seen as a threat, but as a tool—a tool that, when wielded with wisdom and care, has the potential to revolutionize healthcare and improve the lives of providers and patients around the world. So, welcome to the future of healthcare. A future where the power of AI is harnessed to its full potential, where the boundaries between the artificial and the human are blurred, and where the possibilities are as limitless as our collective imagination. Welcome to a journey that I hope will inspire and enlighten you.

Welcome to a narrative that bridges the gap between the artificial and the human, between fear and acceptance, and between the present and the future. This book is an invitation to a journey of discovery and understanding, and that will inspire and enlighten you.

Welcome to the future of healthcare. A future where AI and human intelligence work synergistically to provide better healthcare for all.

Global Chief Nursing Information Officer
Microsoft Health & Life Science Industry
Redmond, WA, USA

Kathleen McGrow

Preface

AI is not the future. It is no longer just an idea or a vision. It has become a reality. In a very short period of just a few years, AI technologies have become present in almost all areas of our daily lives. From online shopping to communicating with your mobile phone provider, from the insurance sector to education, innovative technologies are essential tools that support us in finding the best available information, making better decisions, or tackling complex problems in a fast and effective way. The field of medicine and healthcare is one of the most impressive examples of how AI tools revolutionize the way we think, make decisions, and interact. In virtually all medical disciplines, AI technologies enable in principle more precise diagnoses, personalized treatments, and a preventive focus that allows doctors to intervene early and prevent the onset of adverse health events. The unique ability of AI to make sense of large amounts of data and thereby support human decision-making is key here.

At the same time, particularly in the healthcare sector, concerns have been raised that AI may replace human expertise and erode human relationships. In fields such as radiology and dermatology, computer vision applications are now an integral part of clinical practice and regularly outperform human doctors in single tasks. When it comes to diagnostic accuracy, medical personnel fear not only for their jobs but also for the quality of care they provide to patients. In this regard, it is essential to note that medical treatment encompasses not only accuracy and efficiency but also other key aspects. Healthcare is a human encounter, whereby personal relationships, trust, and responsibility are crucial. How can this work in a setting that increasingly relies on the judgment of machines and reduces the interactions between doctors and patients? How can we avoid disregarding genuinely human competences, such as empathy and contextualizing data with an individual's particular background, as nonessential? In other words, how can we bridge the gap between the apparent advantages of artificial intelligence and human intelligence as an essential part of medical treatment?

This is the fundamental question the book *Bridging Artificial and Human Intelligence: Implementation Strategies and Case Studies in Healthcare* aims to address. By bringing together various perspectives from different academic and professional fields, it offers insights and concrete strategies for fostering the symbiosis between artificial and human intelligence. The book fundamentally challenges the either-or view, following which implementing AI necessarily means replacing human expertise and reducing interpersonal relationships. Instead, it outlines possible pathways for utilizing the best of both worlds in clinical practice. It covers a broad spectrum of topics from the basics of medical informatics in clinical practice to implications for leadership, innovations, as well as ethical and legal aspects. Discussing concrete case studies from various medical fields demonstrates how the symbiosis between human and artificial intelligence can enhance the quality of care, support clinicians in managing data and decision-making, and optimize workflows and documentation.

Osnabrück, Germany Ursula H. Hübner

Greifswald, Germany Giovanni Rubeis

Arlington, TX, USA Marion J. Ball

The original version of the book has been revised with the following corrections in FM. The second foreword by Donald W. Simborg has been removed. Author attribution has been corrected, with Connie W. Delaney replacing Toria Shaw Morawski in a key sentence on page xiii. Additionally, the institutional affiliation for Marion J. Ball has been updated from the Multi-Interprofessional Center for Health Informatics (MICHI) to the Center for Innovation in Health Informatics (CIHI) on page xix. Finally, the names of Long-Chen (Tommy) Li and Yu-Chuan (Jack) Li, previously misrepresented on page xxii, have now been corrected.

Contents

Part I Introduction

1 Introduction: Implementation of Artificial Intelligence for Improving Healthcare 3
Ursula H. Hübner, Giovanni Rubeis, Connie White Delaney, and Marion J. Ball

2 Principles of Artificial Intelligence and Big Data in Healthcare 25
Martin Michalowski, Shan Sun-Mitchell, and Connie White Delaney

3 Human Intelligence and the Caring Imperative 43
Ursula H. Hübner

Part II Innovation and AI Strategies

4 Leadership for Innovation in AI 61
Angela Barron McBride

5 Implementation Science for AI Projects 75
Jan-David Liebe and Ursula H. Hübner

Part III Case Studies

6 Artificial Intelligence in Dermatology 95
Usman Iqbal, Long-Chen (Tommy) Li, and Yu-Chuan (Jack) Li

7 Bridging Artificial Intelligence and Care—Smart Assistive Technologies for Long-Term Care 109
Katrin Lehner and Vera Gallistl-Kassing

8 Generative AI to Assist Physicians 123
Geoffrey Rutledge

9 AI Supporting Nursing Documentation, Workflows and Patient Care 135
Evelyn J. S. Hovenga

Part IV Challenges and Background

10 Navigating Data Diversity and Equity in Healthcare with AI 157
Giovanni Rubeis

11 Regulatory Frameworks for AI: The Legal and Ethical Perspective 169
Volker Lüdemann

12 Ethical Theories for Artificial Intelligence (AI) in Healthcare 189
David L. Meyers and Emily Grime

Part V Conclusions and Outlook

13 Artificial and Human Intelligence: Data as Bridge Builders 213
Ursula H. Hübner, Giovanni Rubeis, and Marion J. Ball

Index 225

About the Authors

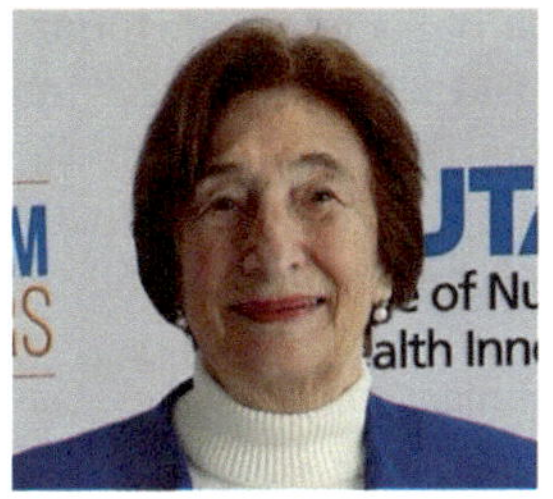

Marion Jokl Ball, EdD, FACMI, FAAN, FIAHSI, FAHIMA, FMLA, FLHIMSS, FCHIME, FIMIA, is the Raj and Indra Nooyi Endowed Distinguished Chair in Bioengineering and Presidential Distinguished Professor and Executive Director of the Center for Innovation in Health Informatics (CIHI) at the University of Texas at Arlington, USA. She is Professor Emerita at Johns Hopkins University in the School of Nursing and has a joint appointment in the Division of Health Sciences Informatics in the Johns Hopkins University School of Medicine. She is a member of the National Academy of Medicine (NAM), has served on the Board of Health on the Net (HON) in Geneva, Switzerland, and was elected as member of the IBM Industry Academy. She is the recipient of both the Morrie Collen award and the François Gremy award. Currently, she works both nationally and internationally on patient safety, nursing informatics, the electronic health record, and enabling technologies as it applies to clinical point of care initiatives.

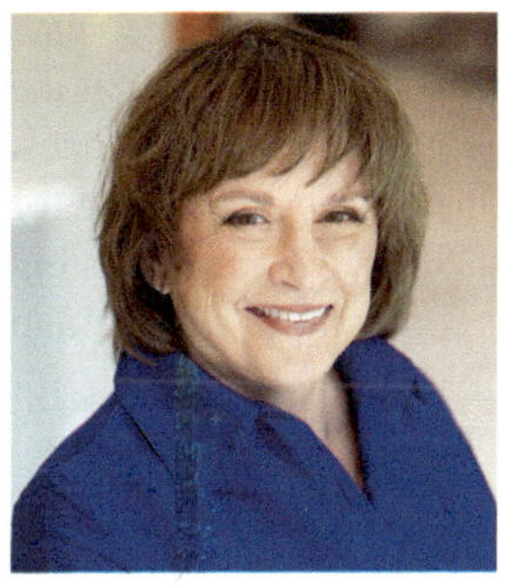

Connie White Delaney, PhD, RN, FACMI, FNAP, FAAN, Professor and Dean, University of Minnesota School of Nursing, is a globally recognized transformation agent in nursing informatics, education, and healthcare innovation. She was among the first to extract code and nursing data from electronic health records, leading to the implementation and US adoption of the Nursing Minimum Data Set, and the development of the Nursing Management Minimum Data Set. She launched the influential Nursing Knowledge Big Data Science

(NKBDS) Conference, now a central platform for advancing nursing informatics research, policy, and practice. She also chairs the American Academy of Nursing's Artificial Intelligence Taskforce, guiding ethical integration of AI into nursing practice.

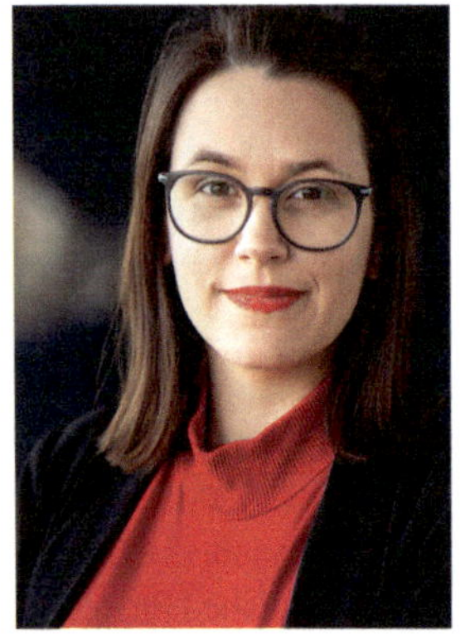

Vera Gallistl-Kassing holds a position as Assistant Professor of Gerontology and Health Research at Karl Landsteiner University of Health Sciences in Krems, Austria. She is a sociologist specializing in health and illness, with a research emphasis on ecological and technological sustainability in the health and care sector. Her work explores how vulnerability and care are constructed across various life stages and institutional contexts, examining the impact of societal transformations—such as digitalization and climate change—on the assessment and negotiation of vulnerability. She studies these topics using quantitative and mixed-methods, with a particular focus on ageing and later life.

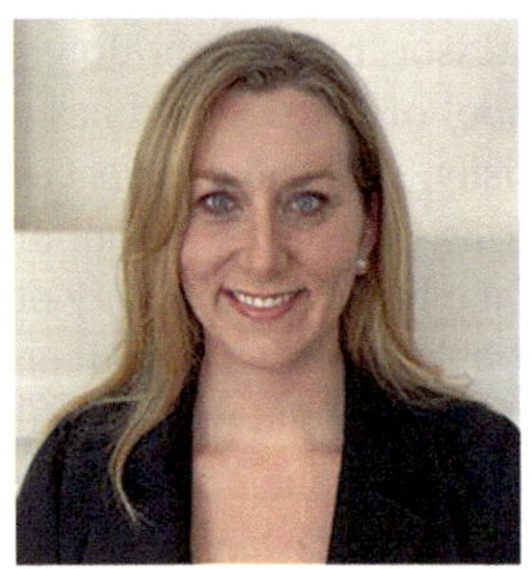

Emily Grime is a seasoned project manager and educator with over 15 years of experience leading global initiatives in healthcare and technology. She holds a doctorate in Bioethics and Health Policy, with a focus on the ethical implications of emerging technologies, including artificial intelligence. Her work bridges practical innovation with ethical responsibility, helping organizations design systems that prioritize equity, transparency, and human dignity. In this book, she explores the evolving role of AI through a lens of ethics, accessibility, and social impact.

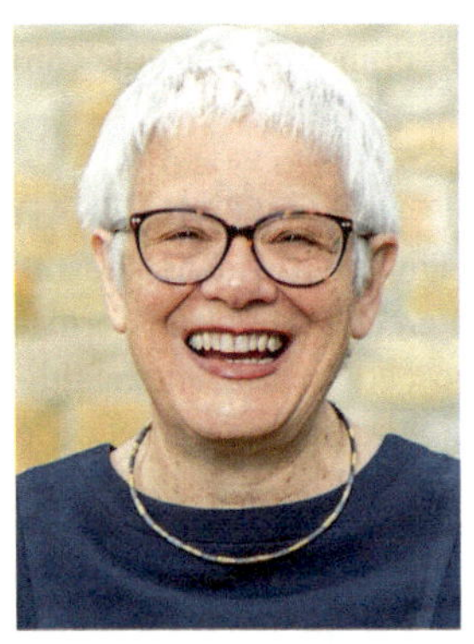

Ursula H. Hübner, PhD, FIAHSI, is Professor of Medical and Health Informatics and Quantitative Methods at the Osnabrück University of Applied Sciences, Germany, where she serves as an associate dean for research, early career, and digitalization at the School of Business Management and Social Sciences. She is founder and co-chair of the research center for Health and Social Informatics. Since her time working for an international computer company in France and Germany, she has been involved in AI research for image analysis in neuroradiology and later for decision support systems in nursing and AI classification systems for chronic wounds. A trained psychologist, she has been interested in the intersection of human behavior and advanced technologies. She has served in various leading roles for scientific national, European, and international medical informatics associations.

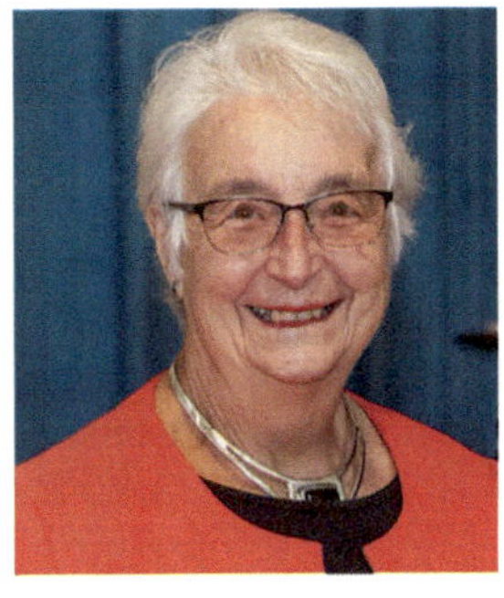

Evelyn J. S. Hovenga, RN, PhD, FACS, FACN, FADHI, FIAHSI, is Honorary Professor in Digital Health at the Australian Catholic University, and consultant. Her exemplary contributions to medicine, particularly in health informatics and digital transformation, have earned her the recognition as a member of the Order of Australia in 2024 and a 2021 Telstra Health recipient of a Brilliant Women in Digital Health award. She is a founding Fellow and life member of the Australasian Digital Health Institute. She is widely published based on research and expertise covering many facets of health informatics, especially standards development, health and nursing terminology, health information governance, electronic health records, including knowledge management, ontology, and semantic interoperability.

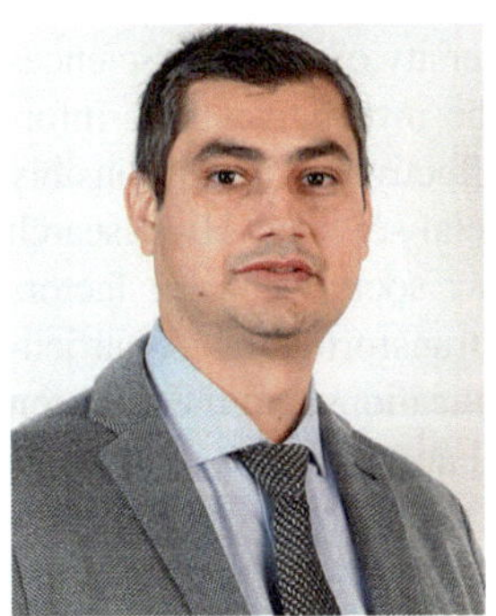

Usman Iqbal, PhD, is a recognized leader in digital health, health informatics, and evidence-based practice. He is a Professor at Bond University, Australia, leads a clinical unit at Gold Coast University Hospital, and is a fellow of several prestigious colleges. He advises global organizations on AI-driven healthcare. His work advances care quality, patient safety, and system performance through technology.

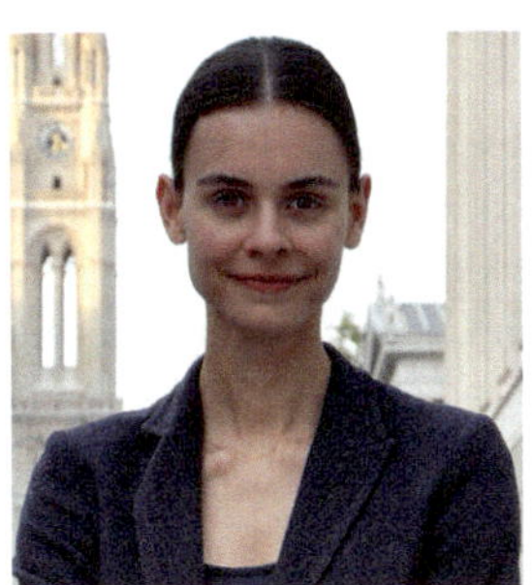

Katrin Lehner is a social gerontologist at the Karl Landsteiner University of Health Science in Krems, Austria, and a PhD student in sociology at the University of Vienna. Her research explores the social construction of age, focusing on practices through which age(ing) is shaped, maintained, and negotiated across diverse societal contexts. With qualitative and participatory research methods, she employs innovative approaches to understand how roles in later life are navigated and redefined in evolving social landscapes. Her current work investigates centenarians' perspectives on the future, experiences of ageing in regions undergoing significant demographic change, and the construction of later life as vulnerable in the context of artificial intelligence.

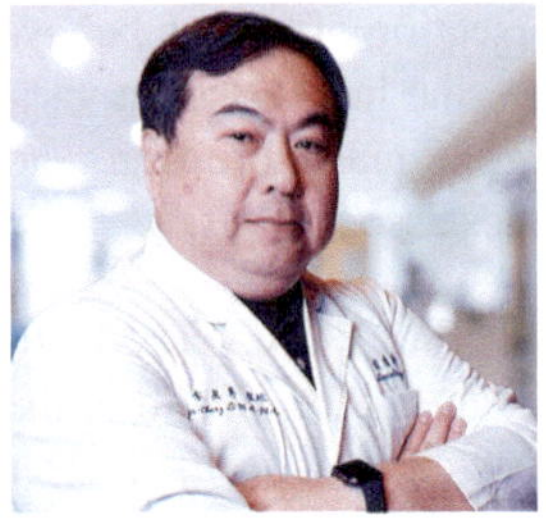

Yu-Chuan (Jack) Li, ranked among the top 2% of scientists worldwide, is a leading expert in AI in medicine. He is a Distinguished Professor at Taipei Medical University, Taiwan, a Fellow of the American College of Medical Informatics and the International Academy of Health Sciences Informatics, and a former President of the International Medical Informatics Association (IMIA).

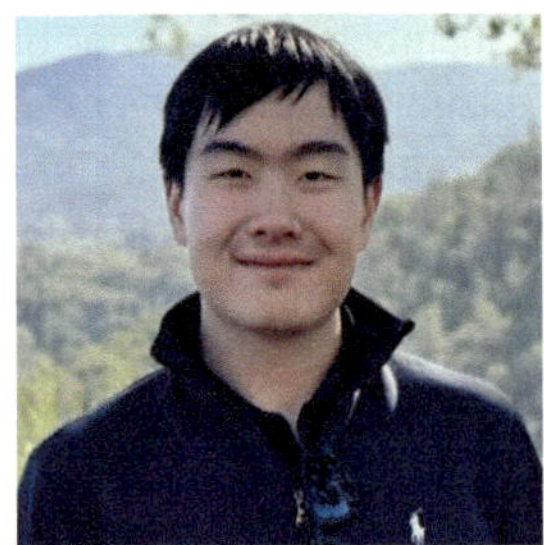

Long-Chen (Tommy) Li is a researcher at Johns Hopkins Medicine, Baltimore, USA, where he leverages artificial intelligence to medical imaging and clinical research.

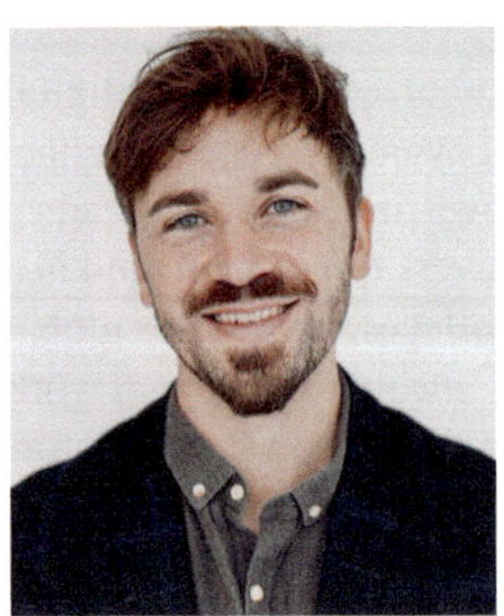

Jan-David Liebe holds the Digitalization Professorship for Digital Society at the University of Applied Sciences Osnabrück, Germany, where he investigates how information technologies can be effectively and responsibly implemented in health and social services. His research addresses the question of how socio-technical factors influence the design of digital transformation. A particular focus is on data-driven applications and the question of how these can be developed and designed in the context of societal requirements, strategic goals, and user-centered needs. Against this background, he examines the role of logic models as a framework for the development, implementation, and evaluation.

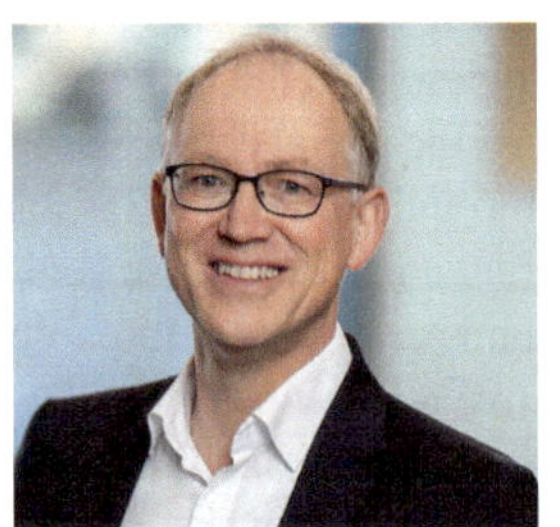

Volker Lüdemann is Professor of Business and Competition Law at Osnabrück University of Applied Sciences, Germany, and Academic Director of the Lower Saxony Data Protection Center. Before entering academia, he held senior legal and executive roles in the automotive industry. His work focuses on data protection and digital transformation law. He advises public bodies and private companies and acts as expert consultant to the German Parliament and state parliaments.

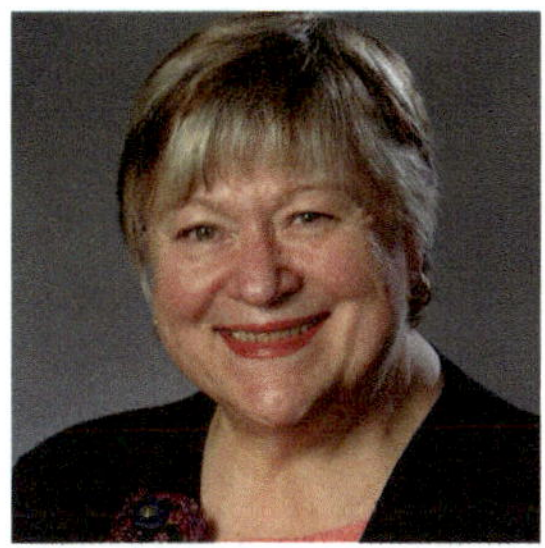

Angela Barron McBride is a Distinguished Professor and University Dean Emerita at Indiana University School of Nursing, USA. In recent years, she has focused her scholarly attention on leadership development, e.g., on how the informatics revolution is changing practice. In 2011, Springer published her book entitled *The Growth and Development of Nurse Leaders*, which won the PROSE Award that year for the category "Nursing and Allied Health"; an expanded second edition debuted in 2020. Her own leadership experience includes serving as president of Sigma Theta Tau International, and as president of the American Academy of Nursing. For her contributions, she has been honored with seven honorary doctorates, elected to the National Academy of Medicine, and designated as a "Living Legend" by the American Academy of Nursing.

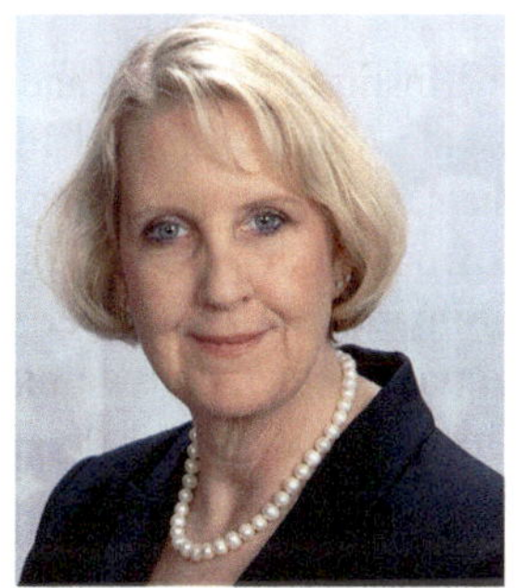

Kathleen McGrow is the Global Chief Nursing Innovation Officer at Microsoft, where she leads strategic initiatives in digital health transformation. Her work focuses on addressing workforce challenges, enhancing patient and provider engagement, and advancing cognitive computing to support a learning health system. She earned her Doctor of Nursing Practice from the University of Maryland, Baltimore. She is a recognized thought leader in the application of artificial intelligence in healthcare, with notable publications including "Foundation Models, Generative AI, and Large Language Models: Essentials for Nursing" and "Implications of Artificial Intelligence for Nurse Managers." Her most recent work is her book, *Empowering Nurses with Technology: A Practical Guide to Nurse Informatics*, published in January 2025.

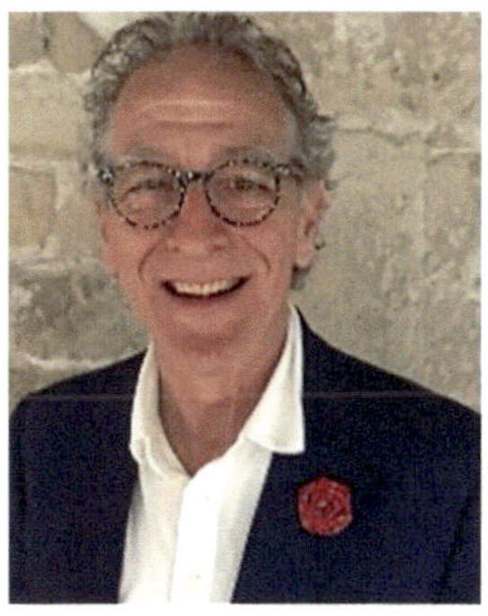

David L. Meyers, MD, MBE, FACEP, HEC-C, is an accomplished physician leader with 40+ years experience as a clinician, healthcare executive, and medical ethicist. Trained in internal medicine and emergency medicine at Cook County Hospital (Chicago) and in bioethics at the Johns Hopkins University Berman Institute of Bioethics, his current interests are largely focused on clinical ethics, ethics in the IT and AI spaces, and advocating for patients through efforts to reduce harm from errors in the course of receiving health care.

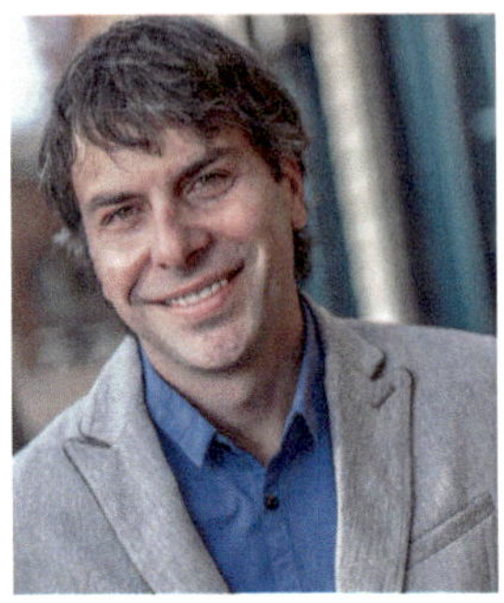

Martin Michalowski is a School of Nursing Foundation Research Professor at the University of Minnesota, USA, where he also serves as Co-Director of the Center for Nursing Informatics and the Digital Health Lab, and he is a co-founder of the Nursing and Artificial Intelligence Leadership Collaborative. He leads interdisciplinary research that applies artificial intelligence methods to clinical decision support, patient engagement, and personalized medicine. He has received several prestigious recognitions, including election as a Senior Member of the Association for the Advancement of Artificial Intelligence (AAAI), Fellow of the American Medical Informatics Association (FAMIA), and Fellow of the International Academy of Health Sciences Informatics (IAHSI). He has published over 100 peer-reviewed articles, secured funding from agencies such as the NSF, NIH, and DARPA, and contributed to patents and startups in health informatics and AI.

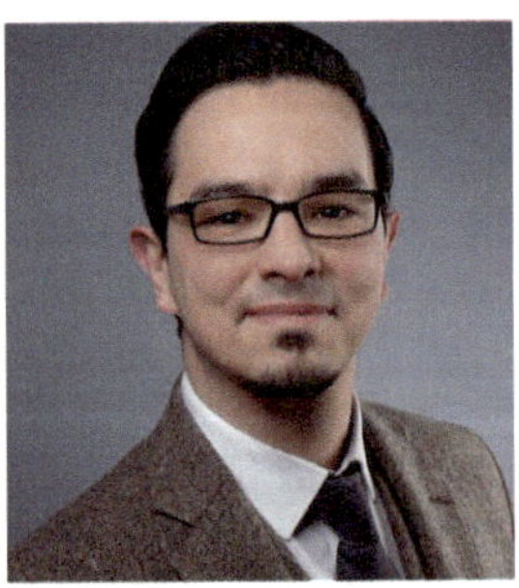

Giovanni Rubeis is head of the Institute of Ethics and History of Medicine at Greifswald Medical School in Germany. After studying at the University of Vienna, Austria, he received his PhD from the University of Tübingen and passed his habilitation at Heidelberg University, Germany. A trained philosopher, he focuses on ethical aspects of artificial intelligence and the digital transformation of healthcare in his research. His recent book *Ethics of Medical AI*, the first comprehensive monograph on the topic, was published by Springer International in 2024.

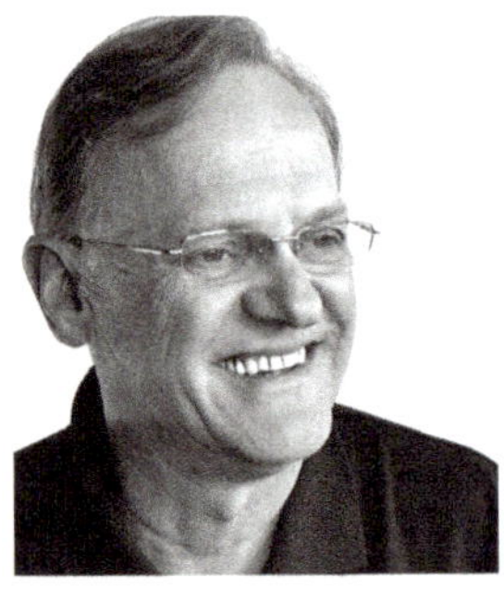

Geoffrey Rutledge founded HealthTap in 2010 to bring health care to mobile devices. He leads HealthTap's doctors and designs their AI tools. He earned his MD at McGill and his PhD in CS/MIS from Stanford. He was NIH-supported faculty at Harvard, Stanford, and UCSD. He created the first version of WebMD.com, led clinical transformation at First Consulting Group, was CMIO at San Mateo Medical Center, and head of product & CMO at Epocrates. He enjoys flying experimental airplanes and hang gliders, scuba diving, cycling, and photography.

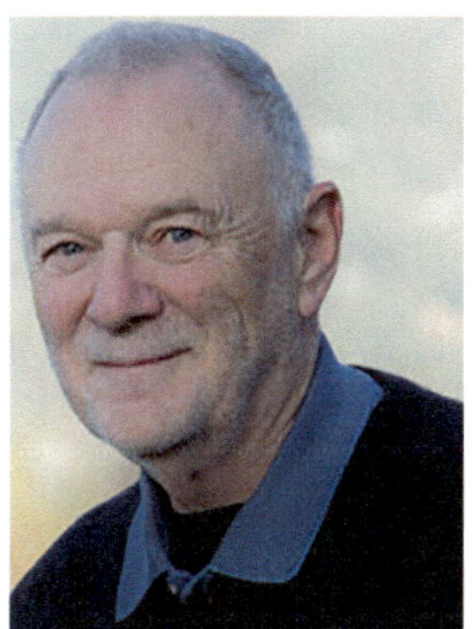

Donald W. Simborg, MD, received his medical education and training from Johns Hopkins School of Medicine. He is a founding member of the American College of Medical Informatic (ACMI) and a Co-founder of HL7. He served as CIO of the University of California San Francisco Medical Center. He has authored among other the book *The Fourth Great Transformation: Creating a New Human Species with AI and Genetic Engineering*, 2024.

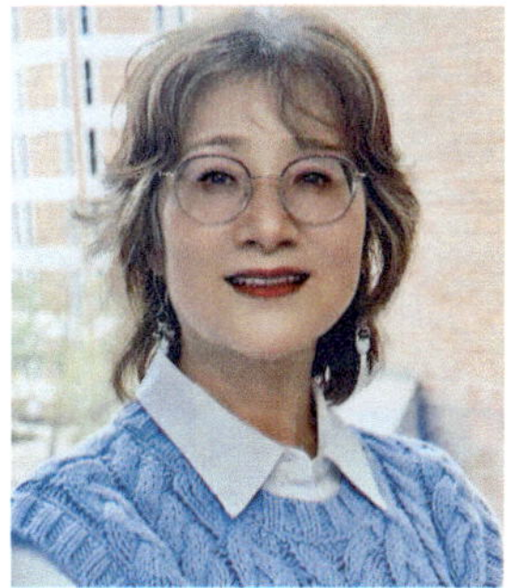

Shan Sun-Mitchell is Professor of statistics in the Department of Mathematics and Co-Director of the Division of Data Science in the College of Science at the University of Texas at Arlington, USA, where she leads interdisciplinary academic programs at both the BS and MS levels. Her research focuses on developing nonparametric statistical methods for complex data structures, with applications in biomedical research and public health, and she actively collaborates with faculty across STEM and health fields. Her prior role as a statistical reviewer at the US FDA shaped her commitment to creating robust, interpretable tools for healthcare decision-making. Her research has been supported by grants from the NIH and NSF, driving the development of innovative statistical frameworks for analyzing physiological signals, clinical trials, and population health data.

Part I
Introduction

Chapter 1
Introduction: Implementation of Artificial Intelligence for Improving Healthcare

Ursula H. Hübner, Giovanni Rubeis, Connie White Delaney, and Marion J. Ball

Learning Objectives
- To understand the embedding of AI in digitalization
- To understand the difference between Artificial and Human Intelligence
- To understand that AI embraces knowledge-based and data-driven approaches
- To understand the roots of AI in medicine and healthcare
- To understand the black box phenomenon
- To describe the promises and risks of AI

Key Terms
- Digitalization
- Artificial intelligence (AI)
- Human Intelligence
- Knowledge-based AI
- Data-driven AI
- Machine Learning
- Prediction models

U. H. Hübner (✉)
School of Business Management and Social Sciences, Osnabrück University of Applied Sciences, Osnabrück, Germany

G. Rubeis
Institut for Ethics and History of Medicine, University Medicine Greifswald, Greifswald, Germany
e-mail: giovanni.rubeis@med.uni-greifswald.de

C. W. Delaney
School of Nursing, University of Minnesota, Minneapolis, MN, USA
e-mail: delaney@umn.edu

M. J. Ball
University of Texas at Arlington, Arlington, TX, USA
e-mail: marion.ball@uta.edu

U. H. Hübner et al. (eds.), *Bridging Artificial and Human Intelligence*, Health Informatics, https://doi.org/10.1007/978-3-032-11938-4_1

- Generative AI
- Explainable AI
- Augmentation of human capacities
- Risks

Summary
This chapter sets the stage of this book introducing the reader to Artificial and Human Intelligence with a special focus on medicine, nursing and healthcare in general. It shows that today's AI is inextricably linked with the achievements of digitalization. Although AI is often used synonymously with machine learning, AI also embraces knowledge-based methods that dominated the early developments in the 1970s. The chapter gives an overview of the spectrum of recent applications, expands on their promise to augment human capacities but also on their intrinsic risks. Bridging Human and Artificial Intelligence requires a good understanding of what both concepts mean and that they represent different realms. However, together they should spur changes and pave the avenue toward the betterment of care provision, patient safety, and patient empowerment.

Introduction: Artificial Intelligence and the Digital Transformation

AI developments are deeply entrenched in the process of digitalization and the digital transformation. AI and digitalization shape each other. Without a massive adoption of electronic health record (EHR) systems hosting digital and structured data, no broad scale analysis of demographic patient data, including individual biomarkers, diagnoses, and treatments, would be possible. AI only started to soar again because of data becoming digitally available. This huge amount of data is usually necessary to train AI models. In turn, it also holds true that the development of clinical AI applications drives the digital transformation. It can motivate healthcare organizations to undertake the efforts of capturing, storing, and providing high quality data in digital form for secondary use. It can propel healthcare organizations to transform themselves into a Learning Health System (LHS), which is the epitome of striving for the improvement of patient services through data. Their analysis—albeit not always AI based—is the engine of an LHS.

The milestones of digitalization (Fig. 1.1), particularly the democratization of information and knowledge,[1] real-time knowledge development, enhanced and enriched visualization of information, cognitive support, connectivity, and mobility [1], could only be reached because of algorithms and statistical methods, and many of them are operating under the roof of AI and machine learning.

[1] By democratizing of information and knowledge we understand the process of opening previously secluded information and knowledge to the broad public via the internet and open access policies.

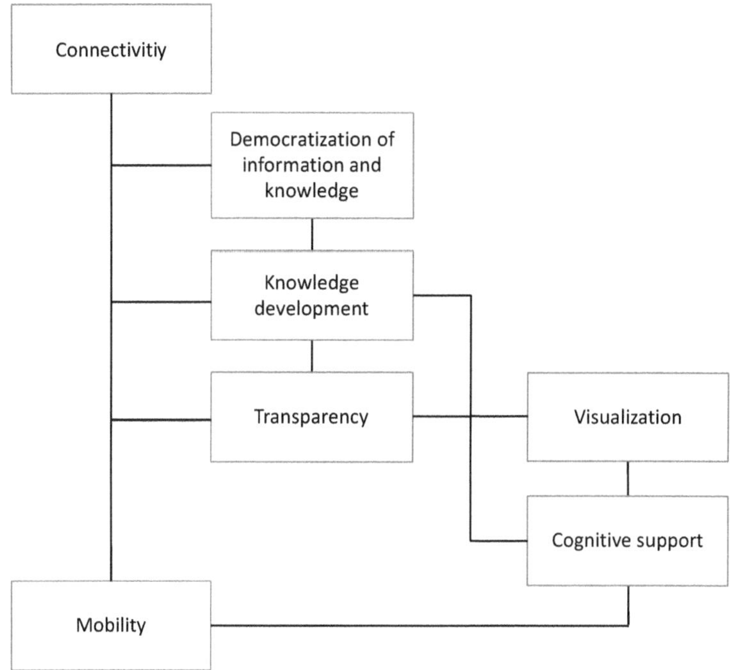

Fig. 1.1 Milestones of digitalization from Hübner et al. [1]. (With permission of the authors)

Knowledge development and cognitive support gain traction through prediction models and Clinical Decision Support Systems (CDSS) while mobility is enhanced through smart sensor and actor interaction when we think about robots. Visualization is advanced through AI generated images and virtual reality. With more cognitive support, e.g., for writing or editing texts, the further enabling of humans and democratization can take place. Finally, the connectivity between humans and machines is raised to a new level through intelligent chatbots and other types of interfaces.

However, there is also a downside. While digitalization opens new doors to obtain greater transparency due to the real time analysis of large amounts of data, deep machine learning models in AI can simultaneously be the reason for less transparency, leading to the black box phenomenon. Without knowing why an AI prediction model came to a certain conclusion, physicians and nurses are not capable of explaining this result to their patients. Therefore, these procedures are further developed as XAI, explainable AI, to achieve greater insights into the mechanisms of deep AI models.

Recent Applications from the Real World in Medicine and Healthcare

As AI innovations are becoming more and more ubiquitous in daily life, these developments have also started shaping the real world of health care processes and outcomes. They may even exert one of the biggest impacts on biomedicine and healthcare compared to other domains.

Good examples are seen in the field of image analysis such as in cardiological imaging [2]. As a scoping review revealed, AI tools performed equally as well as human experts or even exhibited superior diagnostic results. For lung cancer detection, similar findings are seen in the literature. Deep learning methods demonstrated the power to refine lung cancer diagnosis on CT images. They matched human sensitivity and surpassed specificity as a scoping review summarized [3]. In population-wide mammography screening, AI could decrease the radiologist's workload together with enhancing the screening performance [4].

Large language models (LLM) became popular in the early 2020s, entailing applications for various use cases such as workflow improvement to ensure safer patient care. Models could be trained, for example, to identify patterns in patient messages extracted from a patient portal that necessitate an immediate callback. The AI enabled workflow contributed to time reduction before a qualified clinician would see such a message and would induce the appropriate actions [5]. Another use case is knowledge extraction from literature databases such as PubMed. A pipeline starting with retrieving literature on a selected topic, ranking the hits according to a multivariate scheme, and summarizing the top-ranking articles with GPT yielded good results with regard to relevance, quality, and accuracy. It can help clinicians to obtain the latest relevant articles for this topic [6]. AI enabled knowledge extraction features can also be employed for patient education; a case study in diabetic care and the prevention of limb loss demonstrated this very well: The ChatGPT and Pinecone based algorithm extracted knowledge from the NIH National Standards for Diabetes Self-Management Education and could give answers with a very high accuracy rate. The expert reviewed tool was said to be able to enhance health literacy in easy language for patients at risk [7].

All in all, AI based applications in healthcare cover a whole variety of use cases embracing "improvements in operational efficiency, decision support and diagnostic accuracy, advanced interaction and efficient communication, logistical support, workload relief, and ongoing professional development" as a scoping review exhibited [8]. Many individual examples can be found in the literature. Their performance and safe use are to be evaluated in randomized controlled trials and realistic experiments to prove the accuracy, sensitivity, and specificity of their output as well as their added value compared to the usual procedures.

A Short History of AI in Medicine and Healthcare

These developments are possible because AI in medicine and healthcare is not new. It looks back on a long history of significant achievements and ground-breaking innovations. Like in other domains, AI in medicine and healthcare started following a knowledge-based approach where the rules and facts surrounding a topic are specified. Upon querying the system, solutions to the dedicated problems of this topic are inferred from these rules and facts. Already in the 1970s, such a database of pharmaceutical and chemical relations was employed to deduce drug interactions from general pharmacokinetic, pharmacodynamic, or other biochemical relationships [9]. One of the most influential systems that spearheaded AI in medicine was MYCIN as an expert system for infectious disease diagnosis and therapy selection that incorporated a rule acquisition and an explanation component together with the central consultation module for physicians [10].

An entire system of rules and facts can be modeled to become an ontology using specific languages to express reasoning, logical operators, and quantifiers, for example. Rules are often taken from clinical guidelines—in a computer interpretable format—such as in the case of recommending the medication management of multimorbid patients based on goal-oriented input from various clinical guidelines and medical ontologies [11]. Another example shows how the individual target values of HbA1c, when incorporating knowledge from the American Association of Clinical Endocrinologists and American College of Endocrinology, can be proposed and how antidiabetic medication can be recommended, building upon a drug knowledge ontology and a reasoning module. Rules were expressed in a fuzzy way to account for partially true knowledge (degrees of truth) [12]. Both examples originate from recent studies highlighting the fact that knowledge-based approaches representing knowledge in ontologies, semantic web related formalisms, decision tables and rules, logic, and probabilistic models are an active field of research and application [13].

In recent years, AI has been used as a synonym for machine learning (ML), which represents the data-based approach of AI. ML is rooted in the concept of a learning machine proposed by Alan Turing, the construct of a "perceptron", which is an algorithm for binary classification problems from the 1940s and 1950s, and the idea of learning through "backpropagation" in the 1980s [14]. ML was steadily further developed over the next decades, but it was difficult to apply in healthcare due to the lack of large scale digital data. It is now evolving exponentially with the advent and full adoption of electronic health records (EHRs), large radiological image databases (PACS), and other sources of observational health data that are now available and accessible in healthcare. This again exemplifies the role of digitalization for boosting AI in healthcare. In parallel, other crucial trends furnished the health care community with tools: the rise of Deep Learning, i.e., using neural networks with multiple layers [15], the availability of pretrained AI models, and the increase in computational power and new memory concepts. Computing capacity has been provided on a broader scale through High Performance Computing clusters in recent years, while in-memory computing (e.g., SAP HANA in-memory database for hospital information systems) can increase computational performance by mitigating the time loss problem when data are transferred between CPU and memory.

Prominent representatives of machine learning are deep neural networks that leveraged, among others, high performance image classification and generative AI for texts and images. They are built according to a principle that resembles the complex connectivity of neurons in the brain. The examples shown in section "Recent Applications from the Real World in Medicine and Healthcare" made use of these developments. Despite the great interest in AI today, there were times when AI developments stalled, and AI experienced so-called "AI winters". In summary, AI comprises many different methodologies and has seen ups and downs over the last 80 years, now marking an era of obvious successes.

Knowledge-based and machine learning based approaches are sometimes regarded as opposites and adverse worlds: knowledge-based methodologies highlighting evidence derived from randomized controlled trials versus machine learning building upon observational data to develop evidence. However, as both are striving for knowledge, they are complimentary rather than contrary.

What Is Intelligence?

AI embracing the concept of intelligence and thereby referring to human intelligence raises the questions of what "intelligence" is and if artificial and human intelligence share a common core. The two perspectives may also stimulate the discussion on how intelligent human beings can successfully interact with intelligent machines.

"Intelligence" is a psychological construct with a variety of definitions, and it is accompanied by many controversial debates. It has drawn the attention of many scientists in the psychological community since the nineteenth century. Among the various theories, the theory of human cognitive abilities by Cattel, Horn, and Caroll stands out as one of the most and best empirically studied psychometric theories of intelligence. Originally, it embraced the two factors fluid and crystallized intelligence as proposed by Cattel in the 1940s. While fluid intelligence is constituted of inductive and deductive reasoning, crystallized intelligence represents acquired knowledge abilities. Horn added the four components (1) perception and processing, (2) short-term memory, (3) long-term storage and retrieval and (4) speed of processing. Finally, Caroll arranged the results of previous factor analytic work into a hierarchical model composed of three strata of clusters of abilities with the stratum "general intelligence" at the top level [16].

Although general intelligence as the single theoretical construct of intelligence obtains its supports from the fact that many intelligence factors are correlated, there is agreement today that human intelligence is a multidimensional phenomenon [17]. In his book "Frames of mind: the Theory of Multiple Intelligences" from 1983, Gardner postulates the following relatively autonomous human intellectual competencies, i.e., linguistic, musical, spatial, mathematical logical, bodily-kinesthetic and personal intelligence, and speaks about human intelligences in the plural form [18]. However, others such as Sternberg, contend that human intelligent abilities do not appear and work separately. He proposes that creative, analytical, practical, and wisdom-based intellectual approaches collaborate and interact through what he calls "meta intelligence" [19]. Rather than emphasizing different abilities, he argues that it is the purpose for which they are employed that differs. The meta-components orchestrating the cognitive functions are "(1) recognizing the existence of a problem, (2) defining the problem, (3) allocating resources to the solution of the problem, (4) mentally representing the problem, (5) formulating a strategy to solve the problem, (6) monitoring the success of the strategy while it is being used, and (7) evaluating the strategy after it has been employed" [19].

Cognitive psychology that is inherently interested in human information processing looks at the dynamic of problem solving and pursues a process-oriented view, which is a perspective that allows human and computing mechanisms to be made comparable. In an effort to put forward a definition of intelligence that lays the groundwork of a common understanding of human and artificial intelligence, Gignac and Szodorai [17]. define human intelligence as the

> maximal capacity to achieve a novel goal successfully using perceptual-cognitive [processes].

and artificial intelligence as the

> maximal capacity of an artificial system to successfully achieve a novel goal through computational algorithms [17].

These two definitions stress the novelty of the goal as the main criterion distinguishing "novel" from "already known and seen". Computational algorithms embrace all the different approaches of knowledge-based and data-driven AI (machine learning) as presented in section "A Short History of AI in Medicine and Healthcare". Gignac and Szodorai recognize learning as a common feature of both types of intelligence, but they also acknowledge the differences. Harmonizing both perspectives on learning, they offer the definition for human learning

> […] demonstrable change in the probability or intensity of a specific behaviour or behaviour potential, underpinned by neurological processes and cognitive strategies in response to various stimuli.

and of artificial learning in a corresponding manner

> […] demonstrable change in the probability or intensity of a specific response or decision-making potential in an artificial system, underpinned by computational algorithms and data [17].

Not only is machine learning rooted in backpropagation, i.e., a learning concept, but there are other manifestations of learning in computational algorithms and data, such as [20].

- transfer learning, the method to pretrain networks on a large unspecific dataset when the target dataset for solving the problem is rather small
- meta learning, a training procedure for various tasks rather than training a model for a specific task
- autonomous learning, training a model of the world in an unsupervised mode (without labeled data)

Similar to learning, memory span is another a known factor in human intelligence that can also be transferred to artificial intelligence. These shared concepts demonstrate the existence of criteria along human and artificial intelligence that can be expressed, measured, and compared.

They can also highlight the complementarity of both, which is of great practical impact when human and artificial systems interact, intending to achieve better results than they can alone. There are many examples giving evidence of this fact. One study revealed that AI assistance increased the performance of junior readers when assessing radiographic images of knee osteoarthritis. It also improved the interobserver agreement across all readers and experience levels [21]. AI can also help cope with large amounts of data such as in screening programs [4]. In all these instances, AI and humans collaborated with humans having the final say.

The Promise of Augmenting Human Capacity

Acclaimed writer Isaac Asimov who invented the term "robotics", was one of the first to speculate on the potential synergy between human and artificial intelligence. In his essay "Intelligences together" [22], Asimov criticized the dominant trope following which AI will inevitably replace humans. In particular, he contested the assumptions that artificial intelligence is simply a more advanced variation of human intelligence. In his view, both types of intelligence differ from each other. Each has its particular merit: Whereas artificial intelligence may surpass humans in performing one specific task it is designed for, especially where complex data analysis is involved, human intelligence is capable of contextualizing data and viewing the bigger picture. Hence, combining both intelligences would be a far more realistic scenario than replacing one by the other. One could argue that this is especially true in the healthcare domain.

For although AI is discussed and applied to replace humans in other domains such as in industrial production, the value proposition of AI in medicine and healthcare is to augment human capacity rather than to automate processes and outcomes. This particularly holds true whenever decisions and actions have to be made for whom a clinician is personally liable.

Humans are imperfect and their capacity in terms of attention, memory and reaction time is limited due to sensory, cognitive and time constraints. Therefore, the quest is to find ways to counterbalance human deficits with intelligent algorithms. However, also vice versa, AI deficits are to be counterbalanced with human skills and competencies. The underlying scheme portrays a picture of a human-technological team solving complex problems or problems in a shorter timeframe. AI-human-partnering led to an improved diagnostic performance as was shown in a series of studies, such as for the detection of artery occlusions from Computer Tomography Angiography when sensitivity, specificity, and accuracy were improved with AI assistance [23]. In contrast to self-training that increased the diagnostic performance of readers from radiology only, AI support also helped to further improve their diagnostic skills plus the skills of all readers irrespective of their specialty [24]. Apart from diagnostic skills, diagnostic efficiency was also found to increase through significantly decreased reporting times [25]. These examples reflect behavioral enhancements regarding diagnostic outcomes. What they cannot demonstrate are the reasons why these improvements happened and what theoretical underpinning they possess. There is a need for studies to investigate the partnering scenario at a cognitive model level and incorporate theories of decision making and inspecting mediators such as attention and reaction time [26].

Having AI as a team member has raised the fear of the de-professionalization or de-skilling of clinicians when they continuously use AI over time; that would be the opposite of augmentation. This thread, however, was contradicted by clinicians themselves who were experienced AI users. They did not apprehend AI as something that was undermining their profession. Quite the contrary, they regarded the AI recommendation as a complementary view [27]. This rather relaxed attitude may arise from the fact that the clinical decision making of humans differs from that of machines. Whereas clinicians are trained to come to conclusions relying on selected cues from the patients as well as their environments and clinical findings ("ecologically bound"), machine models are typically built on correlations found in very large datasets without necessarily integrating the clinical context ("de-bounding") [26]. Both approaches can end in the same (correct or incorrect) recommendation, but they are distinct on their way toward this end.

In supervised machine learning methods, humans and machines are forced to collaborate as the algorithms require labeled data for training the models, i.e., data seen and classified by humans ("with or without feature X"). When applying these models, further collaboration can take place through feedback given by humans to the machine output. In such case, a mutual augmentation enhances the results in the team scenario.

Beyond the cognitive support provided through AI that is "disembodied", robot "embodied" AI can also act as a partner in medicine and healthcare. One of the best studied fields is robot assisted surgery, which is applied most frequently for radical prostatectomy worldwide. Therefore, this application yields reliable and credible insights into AI enhanced robot assisted surgery [28]. An overview article of AI in this field counted at least ten use cases embracing, among others, AI enabled haptic feedback to warn surgeons about suture breakage, augmented reality guided assistance to identify the tumor and healthy tissue during the nerve sparing phase of the surgery and predicting continence after surgery [28].

There are other possible forms of augmentation that are leveraged through intelligent devices, e.g., insulin pumps, and wearables such as watches. Sensors capturing body signals message them to such devices that can process the data in a smart way. For example, smart insulin pumps can predict the glucose level and adjust the pump activity according to the physical activity level of the patient. This procedure helps type 1 diabetes patients to avoid hypoglycemia induced through physical activity [29] and to augment their independence. Continuous glucose measurements

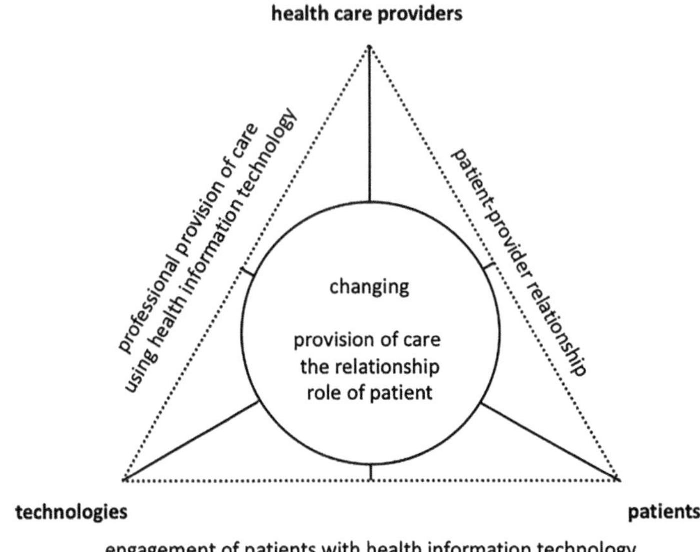

Fig. 1.2 Triade between health care providers, patients and technologies (AI). (Source: own)

feeding their data into prediction models can similarly warn patients via an app about low glucose levels and alert them to take counteractions [30].

The concept of human-AI-partnering to nurture augmentation is in agreement with reality as these examples can manifest. However, the underlying mechanisms that either hinder or facilitate the partnership seem to be poorly understood. The role of trusting AI and developing trust is one of paramount interest. Furthermore, the AI-provider partnership model requires the extension to include the patient who is also interacting with AI (Fig. 1.2).

The Risks of AI

AI does not come without limitations, risks, and threats.

In contrast to knowledge-based AI, machine learning models heavily rely on the data that the models are trained on. Only high-quality data yield high quality AI models. Data quality is an issue in many AI development projects in medicine and healthcare because data quality cannot be taken for granted, particularly in case of secondary data use for research or quality development. The data often stem from Electronic Health Records whose primary focus is clinical documentation and billing. Scrutinizing the quality of data embraces the following criteria:

- accuracy including correctness, timeliness, and validity,
- completeness including relevance and without missing values,
- redundancy including minimality, conciseness, and normalization,

- readability including comprehensibility and clarity,
- accessibility including general availability and technological means for data access,
- consistency including cohesion and without contradictions,
- usefulness including advantage for the users, and
- trust including reliability and data security [31].

As different data sources have to be tapped, the data need to be interoperable to be merged into big data lakes. Interoperability, which is sometimes subsumed by accuracy, first and foremost covers structural and semantic interoperability referring to the same makeup and terminology. When AI models claim generalizability, the data must be representative of the topic the AI model is meant to address, typically originating from multiple clinical centers. For example, when skin lesions are focused on, different skin types and colors must be found in the data set. As many machine learning methods depend on correlations a good amount of variability, i.e. variance in the statistical sense or diversity in a social sense, is necessary to obtain meaningful outcomes. However, there are also characteristics of data that arise from human preprocessing. They mainly refer to the correctness of the data labels that are often—as aforementioned—a result of a manual task succumbed to human errors, prejudices, and predilections. In case data quality is low, AI models are insufficient, possibly biased, and may perpetuate inequalities on a large scale.

Other sources for inadequate AI models are small data size and data imbalance, i.e., unequal amounts of data representing different classes, such as healthy vs. non-healthy. While the impact of data size on model accuracy saturated, data imbalance had a stronger deteriorating effect on model performance [32]. Overfitted models, i.e., having learned from noise and signals very well, and underfitted models, i.e., having learned from too few features, may also pose a threat to their application in daily practice when the model is exposed to new data.

In addition, knowledge-based AI applications may suffer from a lack of quality due to clinical algorithms that are outdated, i.e., the rules and facts. This may happen if the clinical guidelines, as the provenance of the clinical algorithms, are outdated or if the incorporated studies are rather old.

In any such case, data and knowledge flaws are not mere technical problems but demonstrate that quality of care and patient safety are at stake.

Besides biased data that are a risk, the users themselves can be biased when applying technology. Automation bias is defined as the overreliance, under-reliance, or reduced vigilance for errors [26]. If machines fail, overreliance on AI Clinical Decision Support Systems (CDSS) becomes a risky attitude for people to have. While automation bias is not a new phenomenon [33] that is only associated with AI, it has gained new attention as AI applications are increasingly adopted. As confirmed in various studies, overreliance is associated with a high level of trust in the system, a lack of self-confidence, and exerts its power over people in case there is time pressure and a cognitive overload as well as when the task is demanding [33, 34]. The results may be errors of commission, meaning that healthcare professionals follow an incorrect algorithmic decision, or errors of omission, when healthcare professionals do not perform a task because the AI-system did not tell them to [33]. When using an AI CDSS that offered correct and incorrect diagnostic recommendations, clinicians followed a trend of automation bias when they had low diagnostic skills, did not receive special training in this area, and perceived a high benefit for them from this system. Furthermore, profession and gender played a role in accepting wrong machine recommendations [35]. Translating these findings into a practical environment indicates that novices in a field are the most susceptible to incorrect machine output.

A double risk may arise in this context. High performance expectations ascribed to AI-applications and the often perceived superiority when compared to human healthcare professionals might, in some cases, be exaggerated. This is referred to as perfect automation schema [36]. Disappointment of these high-performance expectations may result in a loss of trust in utility of AI-applications in clinical practice. Vice versa, overconfidence in AI performance may lead to automation bias.

These risks corroborate the demand for realistic expectations and good clinical skills on the end of the healthcare professionals to enter the AI-human partnership on equal footing.

Generative AI, appearing as applications for language production as well as the generation of images and other output, bears the risk of false facts. This phenomenon is well described regarding ChatGPT that is known to fabricate DOI numbers. A risk emerges from the errors when people use the tools in an uncritical manner. Out of a large number of clinical decisions on generated wound images, about one third of them deemed the synthetic images to be real. The decisions were made by clinicians with at least a moderate level of knowledge in the field [37].

Deep learning architectures such as convolutional neural networks go along with the disadvantage of not providing insight into the features of the data that most strongly contributed to the output. This is well-known as the black-box phenomenon that may reduce people's confidence and trust in the system. Leaving the clinicians without any explanation about why a decision was made, they are at a loss for an answer not being able to tell their patients the basis of the decision. This may undermine their own credibility as well.

There are procedures to overcome or mitigate the black box. SHAP (SHapley Additive exPlanation) is one of the most known methods from coalitional game theory to exhibit the importance of single features adding to the model output, i.e., the prediction. SHAP is model-agnostic and, therefore, can be applied to a variety of AI procedures, e.g., logistic regression models, non-additive boosted tree models, and transformer natural language processing models [38]. Other means are maps showing the main activation of an algorithm in an image. A well-known representative of this method is Gradient-weighted Class Activation Mapping (Grad-CAM) [39] (Fig. 1.3). It could be shown that the diagnostic performance of domain experts benefits from explainable AI compared to simple AI. Explanations were rendered via heatmaps showing the focus of the algorithms that were juxtaposed with the medical images [40].

Yet another approach questions the imperative of explainability particularly in the context of the patient-provider relationship. Following this view, accuracy of

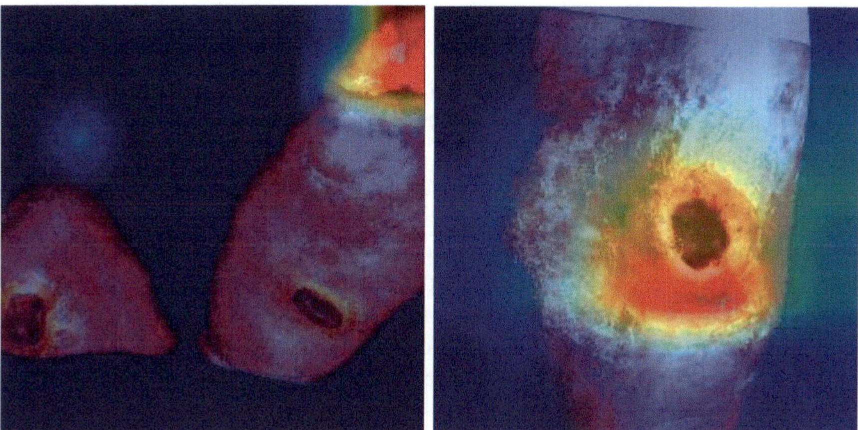

Fig. 1.3 GradCAM results illustrating a wrong (**a** left) and a correct (**b** right) classification of chronic wounds. Whereas in the left image, the activity of the algorithm (red) is outside the wound, the algorithm targets the wound very exactly in the right image

data models is more important than full explainability of how they were developed [41]. Hence, we should focus on the reliability of algorithms, i.e. whether they deliver robust and valid results [42]. This is all the more important since patients are not interested in the technical or statistical intricacies of algorithms, but rather in the clinical implications and their impact on them [43]. Patient-centered explanations should therefore focus on the meaning, risks, and benefits of an AI-supported diagnosis or procedure rather than on the operational logic of algorithms.

Although concerns about the de-professionalization of clinicians are dispelled by findings from some studies, e.g. [27], other studies deliberate the risk of skill decay over time and inappropriate skill development using AI tools. The risk of skill decay may go unnoticed by the clinician and may affect tasks demanding a greater cognitive workload. When applying AI supported systems for training purposes, the question arises as to whether the clinicians are capable of doing without AI support after the training [44]. This matches the finding that well developed clinical skills are good antidotes against automation bias [35]. Both notions speak in favor of lowering the risk through cultivating good clinical qualification programs.

More risks generally emerge when large amounts of sensitive digital data, such as patient data, are captured, stored, processed, and shared. The incidences of privacy breaches and of data security compromises are correlated with the digital availability of data. This holds true for any big data project, but it is particularly the case for AI developments that necessitate large datasets for training the models. Therefore, regulations and frameworks addressing data protection and security to contain these risks are of special interest to AI too. Similarly, accountability and liability are issues of paramount concern.

With these and other risks in mind, organizations and clinicians are ready to implement AI and carry the theory into practice.

From Theory to Practice

The spectrum of AI applications in medicine, nursing, and healthcare requires clinicians to take an active role in their development, implementation, and meaningful use. This refers to the data and knowledge level, socio-technological level, and level of the humans, i.e., the individual healthcare providers and patients as well as their families and friends.

Data and knowledge are at the very heart of any of the healthcare professions. Capturing data is very strongly associated with clinical documentation and patient monitoring that are core tasks of clinicians. Therefore, the clinicians are the ones who must have the final say about data quality in all its aspects. Unsurprisingly, medical associations raised their voice, such as the Society of Critical Care Medicine (SCCM), which established a data science campaign for critical care. This is an area where huge amounts of patient data are produced daily. When striving for large high quality data sets, data need to be harmonized and shared. The Panel on Data Harmonization and Data Sharing of the SCCM set out to define the core data elements as well as their representation, harmonization, and sharing methodology using international health IT standards and terminologies, such as LOINC for health measurements, e.g., lab values, observations, and documents, OMOP (Observational Medical Outcomes Partnership) for standardizing the structure and content as well as HL7 FHIR for sharing data within and across organizations. Their recommendations are construed to incorporate methods capable of dealing with real world data, i.e., messy and imperfect data [45]. Similarly, the Standards for Data Diversity, Inclusivity, and Generalisability (STANDING Together) program, an international collaboration of clinicians, data and AI scientists from universities and industry aims at recommending procedures to assess and declare the limitations and biases of datasets. Their vision is to ensure the transparency of datasets and thereby build a solid ground for developing AI models and scientific knowledge. The recommendations encompass 18 core topics, including those for a dataset summary, the data set identity and access, reasons behind the creation of the dataset, data sampling and aggregation from multiple sources, and ethics and governance. They are meant to help primarily data curators [46]. However, ultimately, they also raise the awareness of clinicians to produce complete and useful datasets when documenting a patient case.

Curating real world data is a task that can be performed semi-automatically by tapping the clinician's knowledge at critical points only. There are systems for automatically assessing data quality in terms of outliers, duplicates, missing values, incompatibilities, and others through statistical analyses that are summarized and provided as a report. Using a clinician developed reference model and ontology of the field of interest, e.g. a disease, this report can be used to curate the dataset. Clinicians are then asked to finally check the curated data [e.g., 47].

At the socio-technological level, questions about how to best fit an AI system into an organization are to be addressed and answered. As it is still a new technology, AI application systems require special attention when introduced into the clinical workflows. As a case study in radiotherapy illustrated, it requires all stakeholders to be mapped, barriers and facilitators to be identified, and an implementation strategy to be developed. The Consolidated Framework for Implementation Research (CFIR) served as a template to describe the context of the implementation as well as to anticipate the barriers and facilitators. Implementation strategies were derived from the Expert Recommendations for Implementing Change (ERIC) strategies employing the CFIR-ERIC Implementation Strategy Matching Tool. Although the concepts of CFIR and ERIC are not tailored to AI key issues, the peculiarities of AI could be identified, and meaningful strategies could be developed. Barriers such as a lack of knowledge and understanding of AI, lacking trust in AI, low confidence in the clinical data used to train AI/machine learning models, lack of stakeholder involvement, the research-clinical practice gap, multidisciplinary collaboration, and the lack of effect measurement were all recognized. The implementation strategies were not specific to one center only but could be utilized by a range of different organizations [48].

The need for AI education and the training of healthcare providers hallmark the human level of transferring AI from theory to practice. This group of persons may be characterized as technological laypersons and non-AI-experts. Therefore, their profile of educational needs to develop AI literacy should differ from that of computer scientists and specialized health informaticians. Laupach and colleagues suggested the TUCAPA scheme of AI literacy, where TU stands for "technological understanding", CA for "critical appraisal", and PA for "practical application" [49], which can serve as an initial grid of understanding clusters of competencies. A similar but extended perspective is presented by Ng and co-workers [50] that incorporates "validation" and "ethics" beyond "technical concepts" and "appraisal", and it embeds AI courses in the field of evidence-based medicine. This perspective is further detailed for different levels of users, i.e., the consumer, translator, and developer. Consumers should be proficient in explaining AI and machine learning, the confusion matrix, limitations and accountability, and levels of evidence, for example. Translators should be familiar with the concepts of supervised and unsupervised model training, information governance, mitigating biases, and clinical endpoints, for example. Developers should possess extended knowledge in training paradigms and methods, synthetic data generation, interpretable engineering, and algorithm analysis [50] (Fig. 1.4).

A scoping review identified three main pillars extracted from the AI curricula. These pillars consisted of "AI use", "interpreting results from AI", and "explaining results from AI" [51]. They partly overlapped with the aforementioned areas and rearranged subtopics slightly differently. For example, "AI use" embraced technological understanding as well as the ethical and legal considerations and limitations, while "interpreting results from AI" referred to medical decision making and data visualization. Finally, "explaining results from AI" covered critical appraisal and added the new topic of communicating with the patient [51].

These three studies—although different in their methodology—arrived at similar competence clusters for clinicians. Obviously, some level of understanding the technology (data, algorithms, models, training, etc.), practical use (interpretation,

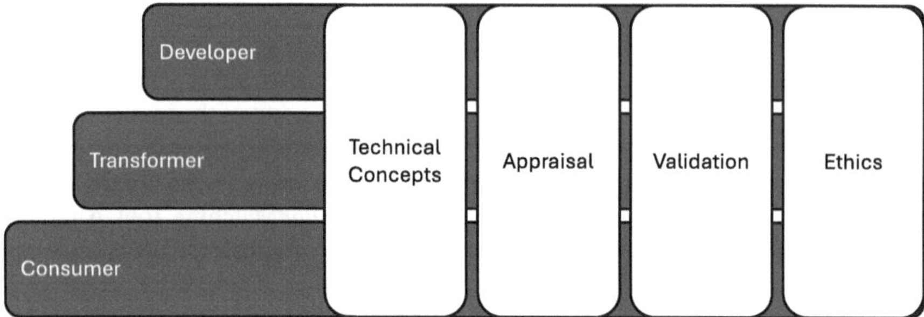

Fig. 1.4 Competency areas and roles of healthcare professionals. (Adapted following Ng et al. [50])

visualization, decision making, explanation, etc.), and a sound capability of appraising AI (performance, biases, limitations, trust, ethics, etc.) are necessary to equip the clinical workforce with the appropriate competencies for the AI age.

Outlook and Conclusions: Bridging Artificial and Human Intelligence

Although both concepts, Artificial and Human Intelligence, share the notion of intelligence, their methods present distinct realms. As the definitions of Gignac and Szodorai [18] reveal, humans harness perceptual-cognitive processes to achieve a novel goal, whereas machines employ computational algorithms. Tikhomirov et al. [26] contend that clinicians apply an ecological filter to the wealth of data while data-driven AI methods exactly live on this wealth of data, reflecting two different approaches to decision making. We therefore have to respect the existence of these two worlds without trying to mingle them or trying to use anthropomorphisms to explain the behavior of AI applications, e.g. "hallucinations" instead of "errors". Having said this, bridging Artificial and Human Intelligence may signify the approximation of these two worlds through a better understanding of the way they attain their output, i.e., diagnoses, recommendations, and conclusions. Such understanding would help clinicians and patients make use of AI models in a synergistic manner and ultimately help incorporate AI enabled applications into human organizations, such as hospitals, clinics, and practices.

Bridging Artificial and Human Intelligence may also be understood as the definition of an arsenal of possible AI methods and applications to benefit patient care because they are leveraged under the umbrella of human oversight. These methods and applications may stem from machine learning and other data-driven concepts or from knowledge-based approaches alike. They may also integrate knowledge from each other mutually.

Bridging Artificial and Human Intelligence also denotes deliberating and agreeing on human regulations and frameworks for avoiding the detrimental and unethical consequences of AI procedures.

In any such case, a novel goal is to be achieved either through Artificial or Human Intelligence. Therefore, the bridging should result in innovation as well as the improvement of patient care and patient well-being. Artificial Intelligence is an innovation in of itself. However, it has to spur changes and pave the avenue toward the betterment of care provision, patient safety, and patient empowerment.

Useful Resources

History and Evolution of Machine Learning: A Timeline. https://www.techtarget.com/whatis/feature/History-and-evolution-of-machine-learning-A-timeline.

Humm BG, Archer P, Bense H, et al. New directions for applied knowledge-based AI and machine learning. Informatik Spektrum. 2023;46:65–78. https://doi.org/10.1007/s00287-022-01513-9, https://link.springer.com/article/10.1007/s00287-022-01513-9.

Rubeis G, Dubbala K, Metzler I. "Democratizing" artificial intelligence in medicine and healthcare: mapping the uses of an elusive term. Front Genet. 2022;13:902542. https://doi.org/10.3389/fgene.2022.902542.

Review Questions

1. How do data-driven AI and digitalization depend on each other?
2. What is the main difference between and what is the main commonality of Human and Artificial Intelligence?
3. What is the difference between knowledge-based and data-driven (machine learning) AI?
4. How did the first AI applications in medicine work?
5. Give an example of how the results of deep neural networks can be explained.
6. Name and explain one promise and one risk of AI.

Answers to Review Questions

1. Data-driven AI—as the name says—requires large amounts of data that became only available with the advent and establishment of electronic patient record systems and other digital sources of data. At the same time, AI models and their applications clearly demonstrate the demand of data which can serve as a driver for processing and storing patient data for secondary use in the sense of a Learning Health System.
2. There are many definitions of Human and Artificial Intelligence. The one this book refers to is the understanding that both concepts describe mechanisms to achieve a novel goal. However, the means are different. While humans make use of perceptual-cognitive processes, machines use computational algorithms.
3. Knowledge-based AI makes use of rules and facts for inference that often originate in clinical guidelines, while machine learning (data-driven AI) needs large data sets to train models that can be used for clinical reasoning.
4. The AI applications in the 1970s followed the knowledge-based approach.

5. Results of deep neural networks can be visualized via Grad-Cam images showing the localization of the main activity of the algorithm.
6. AI promises to augment human capacities which are limited in terms of memory, attention and reaction time. Machines and humans working together in a team can solve complex problems or problems in a shorter timeframe. As several studies show AI-human-partnering led to an improved diagnostic performance. One of the risks of AI is the inclinations of humans to either over-rely or under-rely on machine results or simply ignore them. When AI applications offer incorrect recommendations over-reliance can compromise patient safety and quality of care.

References

1. Hübner UH, Wilson GM, Morawski ST, Ball MJ. Nursing informatics through the lens of interprofessional and global health informatics. In: Hübner UH, Wilson GM, Morawski ST, Ball MJ, editors. Nursing informatics: a health informatics, interprofessional and global perspective. 5th ed. New York: Springer Nature; 2022. p. 3–13.
2. Moradi A, Olanisa OO, Nzeako T, Shahrokhi M, Esfahani E, Fakher N, Khazeei Tabari MA. Revolutionizing cardiac imaging: a scoping review of artificial intelligence in echocardiography, CTA, and cardiac MRI. J Imaging. 2024;10:193. https://doi.org/10.3390/jimaging10080193.
3. Wang TW, Hong JS, Chiu HY, Chao HS, Chen YM, Wu YT. Standalone deep learning versus experts for diagnosis lung cancer on chest computed tomography: a systematic review. Eur Radiol. 2024;34:7397–407. https://doi.org/10.1007/s00330-024-10804-6. Epub 2024 May 22.
4. Lauritzen AD, Lillholm M, Lynge E, Nielsen M, Karssemeijer N, Vejborg I. Early indicators of the impact of using AI in mammography screening for breast cancer. Radiology. 2024;311:e232479. https://doi.org/10.1148/radiol.232479. PMID: 38832880.
5. Yang J, So J, Zhang H, Jones S, Connolly DM, Golding C, Griffes E, Szerencsy AC, Wu TJ, Aphinyanaphongs Y, Major VJ. Development and evaluation of an artificial intelligence-based workflow for the prioritization of patient portal messages. JAMIA Open. 2024;7:ooae078. https://doi.org/10.1093/jamiaopen/ooae078.
6. Li Y, Zhao J, Li M, Dang Y, Yu E, Li J, Sun Z, Hussein U, Wen J, Abdelhameed AM, Mai J, Li S, Yu Y, Hu X, Yang D, Feng J, Li Z, He J, Tao W, Duan T, Lou Y, Li F, Tao C. RefAI: a GPT-powered retrieval-augmented generative tool for biomedical literature recommendation and summarization. J Am Med Inform Assoc. 2024;31:2030–9. https://doi.org/10.1093/jamia/ocae129.
7. Mashatian S, Armstrong DG, Ritter A, Robbins J, Aziz S, Alenabi I, Huo M, Anand T, Tavakolian K. Building trustworthy generative artificial intelligence for diabetes care and limb preservation: a medical knowledge extraction case. J Diabetes Sci Technol. 2024;20:19322968241253568. https://doi.org/10.1177/19322968241253568.
8. Ventura-Silva J, Martins MM, Trindade LL, Faria ADCA, Pereira S, Zuge SS, Ribeiro OMPL. Artificial intelligence in the organization of nursing care: a scoping review. Nurs Rep. 2024;14:2733–45. https://doi.org/10.3390/nursrep14040202.
9. Darvas F, Futó I, Szeredi P. Logic-based program system for predicting drug interactions. Int J Biomed Comput. 1978;9:259–71. https://doi.org/10.1016/0020-7101(78)90025-9.
10. Shortliffe EH, Davis R, Axline SG, Buchanan BG, Green CC, Cohen SN. Computer-based consultations in clinical therapeutics: explanation and rule acquisition capabilities of the MYCIN system. Comput Biomed Res. 1975;8:303–20. https://doi.org/10.1016/0010-4809(75)90009-9.

11. Kogan A, Peleg M, Tu SW, Allon R, Khaitov N, Hochberg I. Towards a goal-oriented methodology for clinical-guideline-based management recommendations for patients with multimorbidity: GoCom and its preliminary evaluation. J Biomed Inform. 2020;112:103587. https://doi.org/10.1016/j.jbi.2020.103587.
12. Chen RC, Jiang HQ, Huang CY, Bau CT. Clinical decision support system for diabetes based on ontology reasoning and TOPSIS analysis. J Healthc Eng. 2017;2017:4307508. https://doi.org/10.1155/2017/4307508. Epub 2017 Oct 26.
13. Riaño D, Peleg M, Ten Teije A. Ten years of knowledge representation for health care (2009–2018): topics, trends, and challenges. Artif Intell Med. 2019;100:101713. https://doi.org/10.1016/j.artmed.2019.101713.
14. Michelucci U. Machine learning: history and terminology. In: Fundamental mathematical concepts for machine learning in science. Cham: Springer; 2024. https://doi.org/10.1007/978-3-031-56431-4_2.
15. Padilha França R, Borges Monteiro AC, Arthur R, Iano Y. Chapter 3 – An overview of deep learning in big data, image, and signal processing in the modern digital age. In: Piuri V, Raj S, Genovese A, Srivastava R, editors. Hybrid computational intelligence for pattern analysis, trends in deep learning methodologies. New York: Academic; 2021. p. 63–87. https://doi.org/10.1016/B978-0-12-822226-3.00003-9.
16. Flanagan DP, Dixon SG. The Cattell-Horn-Carroll theory of cognitive abilities. In: Encyclopedia of special education: a reference for the education of children, adolescents, and adults with disabilities and other exceptional individuals. Wiley online library; 2014. https://doi.org/10.1002/9781118660584.ese0431.
17. Gignac GE, Szodorai ET. Defining intelligence: bridging the gap between human and artificial perspectives. Intelligence. 2024;104:101832. https://doi.org/10.1016/j.intell.2024.101832.
18. Gardener EH. Frames of mind frames of mind: the theory of multiple intelligences. 1st ed. New York: Basic Books; 2011.
19. Sternberg RJ, Glaveanu V, Karami S, Kaufman JC, Phillipson SN, Preiss DD. Meta-intelligence: understanding, control, and interactivity between creative, analytical, practical, and wisdom-based approaches in problem solving. J Intelligence. 2021;9:19. https://doi.org/10.3390/jintelligence9020019.
20. Zhu S, Yu T, Xu T, Chen H, Dustdar S, Gigan S, Gunduz D, Hossain E, Jin Y, Lin F, et al. Intelligent computing: the latest advances, challenges, and future. Intell Comput. 2023;2:0006. https://doi.org/10.34133/icomputing.0006.
21. Brejnebøl MW, Lenskjold A, Ziegeler K, Ruitenbeek H, Müller FC, Nybing JU, Visser JJ, Schiphouwer LM, Jasper J, Bashian B, Cao H, Muellner M, Dahlmann SA, Radev DI, Ganestam A, Nielsen CT, Stroemmen CU, Oei EHG, Hermann KA, Boesen M. Interobserver agreement and performance of concurrent AI assistance for radiographic evaluation of knee osteoarthritis. Radiology. 2024;312:e233341. https://doi.org/10.1148/radiol.233341.
22. Asimov I. Intelligences together. In: Asimov I, editor. The dangers of intelligence and other science essays. Houghton Mifflin Company: Boston; 1986. p. 92–4.
23. Li K, Yang Y, Yang Y, Li Q, Jiao L, Chen T, Guo D. Added value of artificial intelligence solutions for arterial stenosis detection on head and neck CT angiography: a randomized crossover multi-reader multi-case study. Diagn Interv Imaging. 2024;S2211-5684:00169–4. https://doi.org/10.1016/j.diii.2024.07.008.
24. Lee SE, Kim HJ, Jung HK, Jung JH, Jeon JH, Lee JH, Hong H, Lee EJ, Kim D, Kwak JY. Improving the diagnostic performance of inexperienced readers for thyroid nodules through digital self-learning and artificial intelligence assistance. Front Endocrinol (Lausanne). 2024;15:1372397. https://doi.org/10.3389/fendo.2024.1372397. Erratum in: Front Endocrinol (Lausanne) 2024 Sep 02;15:1466012. https://doi.org/10.3389/fendo.2024.1466012.
25. Peters S, Kellermann G, Watkinson J, Gartner F, Huhndorf M, Stürner K, Jansen O, Larsen N. AI supported detection of cerebral multiple sclerosis lesions decreases radiologic reporting times. Eur J Radiol. 2024;178:111638. https://doi.org/10.1016/j.ejrad.2024.111638.

26. Tikhomirov L, Semmler C, McCradden M, Searston R, Ghassemi M, Oakden-Rayner L. Medical artificial intelligence for clinicians: the lost cognitive perspective. Lancet Digit Health. 2024;6:e589–94. https://doi.org/10.1016/S2589-7500(24)00095-5. PMID: 39059890.
27. Johansson JV, Engström E. Humans think outside the pixels' – radiologists' perceptions of using artificial intelligence for breast cancer detection in mammography screening in a clinical setting. Health Informatics J. 2024;30:14604582241275020. https://doi.org/10.1177/14604582241275020. PMID: 39155239.
28. Carbin DD, Shah A, Kusuma VRM. Artificial intelligence in robot-assisted radical prostatectomy: where do we stand today? J Robot Surg. 2024;18:404. https://doi.org/10.1007/s11701-024-02143-x.
29. Moser O, Zaharieva DP, Adolfsson P, Battelino T, Bracken RM, Buckingham BA, Danne T, Davis EA, Dovč K, Forlenza GP, Gillard P, Hofer SE, Hovorka R, Jacobs PG, Mader JK, Mathieu C, Nørgaard K, Oliver NS, O'Neal DN, Pemberton J, Rabasa-Lhoret R, Sherr JL, Sourij H, Tauschmann M, Yardley JE, Riddell MC. The use of automated insulin delivery around physical activity and exercise in type 1 diabetes: a position statement of the European Association for the Study of Diabetes (EASD) and the International Society for Pediatric and Adolescent Diabetes (ISPAD). Diabetologia. 2025;68:255–80. https://doi.org/10.1007/s00125-024-06308-z.
30. Herrero P, Andorrà M, Babion N, Bos H, Koehler M, Klopfenstein Y, Leppäaho E, Lustenberger P, Peak A, Ringemann C, Glatzer T. Enhancing the capabilities of continuous glucose monitoring with a predictive app. J Diabetes Sci Technol. 2024;18:1014–26. https://doi.org/10.1177/19322968241267818.
31. Batini C, Scannapieco M. Data and information quality – dimensions, principles and techniques. Cham: Springer; 2016. https://doi.org/10.1007/978-3-319-24106-7.
32. Davidian M, Lahav A, Joshua BZ, Wand O, Lurie Y, Mark S. Exploring the interplay of dataset size and imbalance on CNN performance in healthcare: using X-rays to identify COVID-19 patients. Diagnostics (Basel). 2024;14:1727. https://doi.org/10.3390/diagnostics14161727.
33. Goddard K, Roudsari A, Wyatt JC. Automation bias: a systematic review of frequency, effect mediators, and mitigators. J Am Med Inform Assoc. 2012;19:121–7. https://doi.org/10.1136/amiajnl-2011-000089.
34. Bond RR, Novotny T, Andrsova I, Koc L, Sisakova M, Finlay D, Guldenring D, McLaughlinc J, Peace A, McGilligan V, Leslie SJ, Wang H, Malik M. Automation bias in medicine: the influence of automated diagnoses on interpreter accuracy and uncertainty when reading electrocardiograms. J Electrocardiol. 2018;51:S6–S11. https://doi.org/10.1016/j.jelectrocard.2018.08.007.
35. Kücking F, Hübner U, Przysucha M, Hannemann N, Kutza JO, Moelleken M, Erfurt-Berge C, Dissemond J, Babitsch B, Busch D. Automation bias in AI-decision support: results from an empirical study. Stud Health Technol Inform. 2024;317:298–304. https://doi.org/10.3233/SHTI240871.
36. Rieger T, Roesler E, Manzey D. Challenging presumed technological superiority when working with (artificial) colleagues. Sci Rep. 2022;12:3768. https://doi.org/10.1038/s41598-022-07808-x.
37. Malihi L, Hübner U, Richter ML, Moelleken M, Przysucha M, Busch D, Heggemann J, Hafer G, Wiemeyer S, Heidemann G, Dissemond J, Erfurt-Berge C, Barkhau C, Hendriks A, Hüsers J. Can synthetic images improve CNN performance in wound image classification? Stud Health Technol Inform. 2023;302:927–31. https://doi.org/10.3233/SHTI230311.
38. Molnar C. Interpretable machine learning. A guide for making black box models explainable. 2nd ed. Munich: Christoph Molnar; 2024. Available from: https://christophm.github.io/interpretable-ml-book.
39. Selvaraju RR, Cogswell M, Das A, Vedantam R, Parikh D, Batra D. Grad-CAM: visual explanations from deep networks via gradient-based localization. In: 2017 IEEE International Conference on Computer Vision (ICCV), Venice, Italy. IEEE; 2017. p. 618–26. https://doi.org/10.1109/ICCV.2017.74.

40. Senoner J, Schallmoser S, Kratzwald B, Feuerriegel S, Netland T. Explainable AI improves task performance in human-AI collaboration. Sci Rep. 2024;14:31150. https://doi.org/10.1038/s41598-024-82501-9.
41. London AJ. Artificial intelligence and black-box medical decisions: accuracy versus explainability. Hast Cent Rep. 2019;15:49.
42. Durán JM, Jongsma KR. Who is afraid of black box algorithms? On the epistemological and ethical basis of trust in medical AI. J Med Ethics. 2021;47:medethics-2020-106820. https://doi.org/10.1136/medethics-2020-106820.
43. Rubeis G. Ethis of medical AI. Cham: Springer; 2024.
44. Macnamara BN, Berber I, Çavuşoğlu MC, Krupinski EA, Nallapareddy N, Nelson NE, Smith PJ, Wilson-Delfosse AL, Ray S. Does using artificial intelligence assistance accelerate skill decay and hinder skill development without performers' awareness? Cogn Res Princ Implic. 2024;9:46. https://doi.org/10.1186/s41235-024-00572-8.
45. Heavner SF, Kumar VK, Anderson W, Al-Hakim T, Dasher P, Armaignac DL, Clermont G, Cobb JP, Manion S, Remy KE, Reuter-Rice K, Haendel M. Critical data for critical care: a primer on leveraging electronic health record data for research from Society of Critical Care Medicine's panel on data sharing and harmonization. Crit Care Explor. 2024;6:e1179. https://doi.org/10.1097/CCE.0000000000001179.
46. Alderman JE, Palmer J, Laws E, McCradden MD, Ordish J, Ghassemi M, et al. Tackling algorithmic bias and promoting transparency in health datasets: the STANDING together consensus recommendations. Lancet Digit Health. 2025;7:e64–88. https://doi.org/10.1016/S2589-7500(24)00224-3.
47. Pezoulas VC, Kourou KD, Kalatzis F, Exarchos TP, Venetsanopoulou A, Zampeli E, Gandolfo S, Skopouli F, De Vita S, Tzioufas AG, Fotiadis DI. Medical data quality assessment: on the development of an automated framework for medical data curation. Comput Biol Med. 2019;107:270–83. https://doi.org/10.1016/j.compbiomed.2019.03.001.
48. Swart R, Boersma L, Fijten R, van Elmpt W, Cremers P, Jacobs MJG. Implementation strategy for artificial intelligence in radiotherapy: can implementation science help? JCO Clin Cancer Inform. 2024;8:e2400101. https://doi.org/10.1200/CCI.24.00101.
49. Laupichler MC, Aster A, Haverkamp N, Raupach T. Development of the "scale for the assessment of non-experts' AI literacy" – an exploratory factor analysis. Comput. Hum. Behav. Rep. 2023;12:100338. https://doi.org/10.1016/j.chbr.2023.100338.
50. Ng FYC, Thirunavukarasu AJ, Cheng H, Tan TF, Gutierrez L, Lan Y, Ong JCL, Chong YS, Ngiam KY, Ho D, Wong TY, Kwek K, Doshi-Velez F, Lucey C, Coffman T, Ting DSW. Artificial intelligence education: an evidence-based medicine approach for consumers, translators, and developers. Cell Rep Med. 2023;4:101230. https://doi.org/10.1016/j.xcrm.2023.101230.
51. Charow R, Jeyakumar T, Younus S, Dolatabadi E, Salhia M, Al-Mouaswas D, et al. Artificial intelligence education programs for health care professionals: scoping review. JMIR Med Educ. 2021;7:e31043. https://doi.org/10.2196/31043.

Chapter 2
Principles of Artificial Intelligence and Big Data in Healthcare

Martin Michalowski, Shan Sun-Mitchell, and Connie White Delaney

Learning Objectives

- To understand foundational concepts and definitions related to AI and Big Data.
- To differentiate between rule-based and data-driven AI.
- To identify the distinctions and applications of embodied versus disembodied AI.
- To distinguish between statistical methods and deep learning techniques.
- To describe generative AI and its relevance to healthcare.
- To discuss the importance of data, algorithms, and explainability in data-driven AI.
- To recognize ethical implications and the importance of human oversight in AI applications.

Key Terms

Here are some examples:

- Artificial intelligence (AI)
- Big data
- Rule-based AI
- Data-driven AI
- Embodied AI

M. Michalowski · C. W. Delaney (✉)
School of Nursing, University of Minnesota, Minneapolis, MN, USA
e-mail: delaney@umn.edu

S. Sun-Mitchell
Department of Mathematics, University of Texas at Arlington, Arlington, TX, USA

U. H. Hübner et al. (eds.), *Bridging Artificial and Human Intelligence*, Health Informatics, https://doi.org/10.1007/978-3-032-11938-4_2

- Disembodied AI
- Statistical methods
- Deep learning
- Generative AI
- Explainability
- Ethical AI

Summary
Artificial Intelligence (AI) and Big Data have emerged as transformative forces in modern healthcare, redefining how clinical data is interpreted, decisions are made, care is delivered, and health of individuals, families, and communities is advanced. This chapter includes the historical evolution of AI in healthcare, clarifies foundational definitions, compares rule-based and data-driven approaches, differentiates embodied and disembodied systems, contrasts statistical methods with deep learning, introduces generative AI, explores algorithms, data quality, and explainability in depth, discusses ethical considerations and human oversight, presents real-world use cases, and concludes with future directions.

Introduction

Artificial Intelligence (AI) and Big Data have emerged as transformative forces in modern healthcare, redefining how clinical data are interpreted, decisions made, care delivered, and the health of individuals, families, and communities promoted. These technologies offer powerful tools to address longstanding challenges in health and healthcare, including diagnostic errors, inefficiencies in care delivery, underutilization of patient data, and threats to the health of the public. By analyzing complex datasets with unprecedented speed and accuracy, AI enables predictive insights, personalized treatment plans, enhanced decision support for clinicians, protecting public health and advancing population well-being [3, 6].

At the core of AI's integration into healthcare are several key methodologies: rule-based systems that use structured logic to guide clinical decisions; and data-driven models, especially those based on machine learning (ML) and deep learning (DL), that can learn patterns and associations from vast and diverse datasets. Embodied AI systems, such as surgical robots, have revolutionized procedural medicine, while disembodied AI applications, like clinical decision support systems (CDSS) embedded in electronic health records (EHRs), assist clinicians in diagnosis and risk stratification without physical presence [29]. Moreover, generative AI is beginning to reshape areas such as medical image synthesis, drug discovery, and clinician/patient relationships [15].

However, the power of these technologies also brings significant ethical, technical, and regulatory challenges. Data privacy, algorithmic bias, explainability, and accountability are central to ongoing debates about the responsible use of AI in healthcare [1, 25]. Health care providers must balance the potential for AI to improve patient outcomes with the need to ensure equitable, transparent, patient-centered, whole-person care. Human oversight remains critical— for clinical accountability as well as fostering trust in AI-assisted care.

The sections that follow provide a structured roadmap through the evolution of AI in healthcare—defining core concepts, distinguishing approaches, examining key ethical and technical considerations, and illustrating practical applications and future directions.

Historical Context of AI in Healthcare

Artificial Intelligence (AI) has a long history in general (Fig. 2.1), and in healthcare dating back to the 1970s, when early expert systems designed for diagnostic purposes were developed. One of the first notable AI systems was MYCIN, which assisted physicians by recommending antibiotics based on patient symptoms and laboratory results [22]. These early rule-based systems operated on explicitly programmed expert knowledge and demonstrated the potential of AI to aid clinical decision-making.

The late 1990s and early 2000s saw a pivot toward data-driven learning as electronic health records (EHRs) became ubiquitous. Machine-learning classifiers and ensemble methods leveraged structured laboratory and claims data to predict outcomes such as hospital readmission and sepsis risk [3]. A major inflection occurred in the 2010s with graphics-processing-unit (GPU)–accelerated deep learning. Convolutional neural networks (CNNs) demonstrated radiologist-level accuracy in image classification, influencing disciplines from radiology and dermatology to pathology [6].

The introduction of transformer architectures and self-attention [24] enabled large-scale language and vision models. Foundation models such as BioBERT and Med-PaLM leveraged unsupervised pre-training on biomedical corpora, achieving near-expert-level performance on question-answering tasks. In parallel, Generative Adversarial Networks (GANs) and diffusion models began producing high-fidelity synthetic medical images, helping address data scarcity, class imbalance, and privacy preservation in training data sets. These advances set the stage for multimodal, generative, and conversational AI tools now entering clinical trials. Together, these waves—from expert systems to deep, generative architectures—illustrate a trajectory of increasing data-dependency, model complexity, and clinical impact while amplifying the need for transparency and regulation.

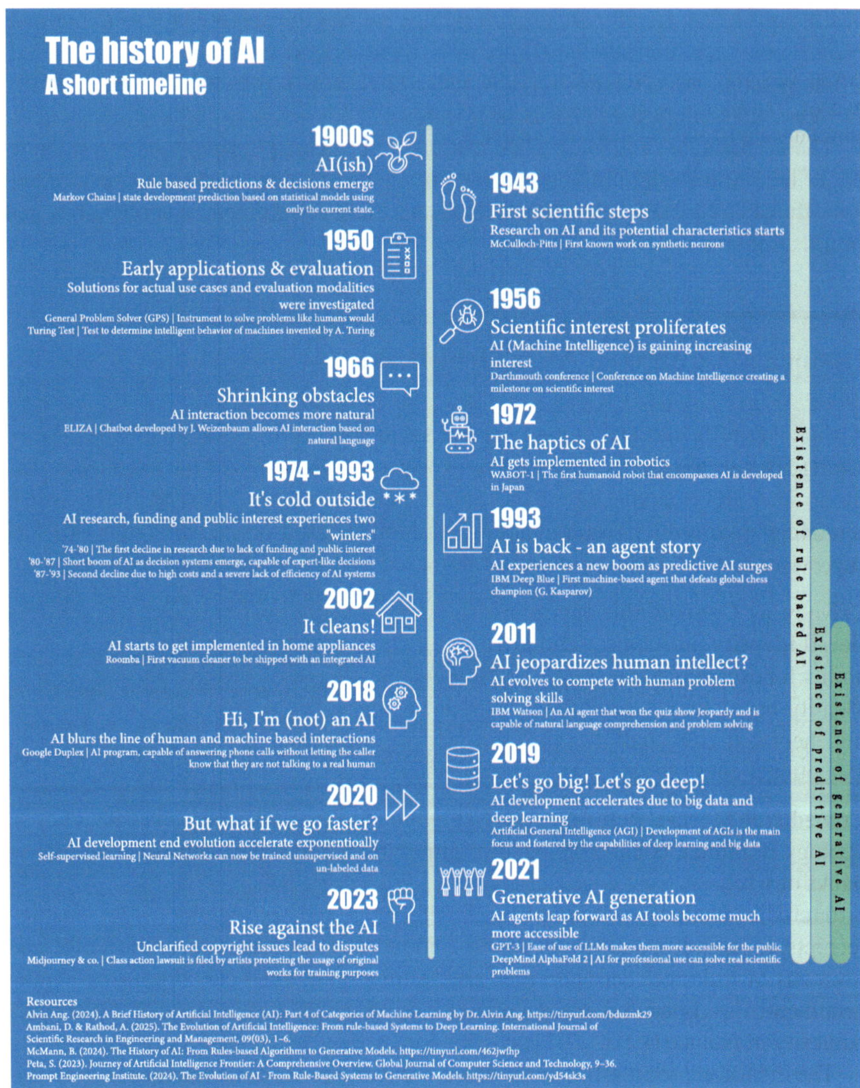

Fig. 2.1 Short history of AI—timeline

Definitions and Core Concepts

Artificial Intelligence (AI) encompasses various computational methods and algorithms designed to perform tasks traditionally requiring human intelligence, such as learning from data, recognizing patterns, and making informed decisions [29]. Central to AI's utility in healthcare is its ability to process and interpret complex data swiftly and accurately. AI in healthcare broadly includes machine learning

(ML), deep learning (DL), natural language processing (NLP), computer vision, and robotics each offering distinct capabilities and applications.

Machine learning, a subset of AI, refers to algorithms that learn patterns from data and make predictions or decisions without explicit programming. ML can be supervised, unsupervised, or reinforcement learning, depending on the presence and role of labeled data and the learning approach used [3]. Deep learning, a specialized branch of ML, employs artificial neural networks composed of multiple layers. This hierarchical structure allows DL models to capture complex nonlinear relationships within large, unstructured datasets, making it particularly suited for analyzing medical images, genomic data, and electronic health records [6]. Natural language processing enables machines to understand, interpret, and generate human language, making it essential for tasks like clinical documentation analysis and voice-enabled interfaces [26, 27]. Computer vision allows AI systems to extract meaningful information from medical images, supporting diagnostics and image-guided procedures [6, 13]. Big Data in healthcare refers to datasets of substantial volume, velocity, variety, and complexity—such as electronic health records (EHRs), medical imaging archives, genomic sequences, and data from wearable sensors. These datasets often exceed traditional analytical capabilities and require advanced computational tools. AI techniques, particularly ML and DL, are essential for extracting meaningful insights from Big Data, driving advances in precision medicine, early disease detection, and population health management [23].

Rule-Based Versus Data-Driven AI

Rule-based AI systems depend on explicit instructions or rules manually coded by human experts, providing logical pathways for decision-making processes. A classic example of rule-based AI is the traditional Clinical Decision Support System (CDSS), which guides clinicians by applying established clinical guidelines or best practices to individual patient scenarios. These systems utilize clearly defined criteria, such as symptom checklists or decision trees, enabling straightforward and transparent decision-making [22]. While effective for straightforward clinical scenarios with well-established guidelines, rule-based systems are inherently limited by their inability to adapt or evolve without significant manual intervention and updates.

Data-driven AI, conversely, relies on machine learning algorithms that identify patterns directly from large and complex datasets. These approaches learn continuously, refining their predictive accuracy and adaptability as more data becomes available. Data-driven methods include supervised learning, where models are trained on labeled datasets; unsupervised learning, which discovers hidden patterns in unlabeled data; and reinforcement learning, where models improve through feedback from sequential decision outcomes [3].

In healthcare, data-driven AI has been highly effective in personalized medicine, predictive analytics, and diagnostics—especially in fields like oncology, radiology, and cardiology, where predictive accuracy is vital for patient outcomes.

An important distinction between these approaches is their transparency and explainability. Rule-based systems typically offer high transparency, making it easier for clinicians to understand and trust their recommendations. Conversely, data-driven methods, especially deep learning, can be perceived as "black boxes"due to their complex and opaque decision-making processes. This is primarily because these models involve thousands—or even millions—of parameters, making it difficult to trace how specific inputs contribute to outputs. This opacity has prompted significant research into Explainable AI (XAI) techniques to improve transparency and trust in data-driven healthcare applications [1].

Rule-based AI employs explicit, expert-curated logic to produce determinate recommendations, whereas data-driven AI infers patterns from historical data. Hybrid AI systems integrate elements of both rule-based and data-driven approaches, using predefined rules for safety and interpretability while allowing machine learning components to adapt to new data and improve performance over time. Between these poles lies a growing class of hybrid systems that combine rules for safety with machine-learning models for adaptability. A widely cited example is the Targeted Real-time Early Warning System (TREWS) for sepsis at Johns Hopkins: strict physiological thresholds trigger the alert (rule-based), while an embedded gradient-boosting model continuously recalibrates individual risk scores using streaming vitals and laboratory data [12]. Hybrid designs leverage the transparency of rules to preserve clinician trust, yet still realize performance gains from data-driven components—illustrating that rule-based and learning-based AI should be seen as a continuum rather than mutually exclusive categories. This blended approach is increasingly viewed as a path toward both innovation and accountability in clinical AI.

Embodied and Disembodied AI

Embodied AI refers to systems in which artificial intelligence is integrated into physical entities or robotic platforms capable of interacting physically with their environment. In healthcare, embodied AI includes robotic surgical assistants, robotic rehabilitation devices, and robotic patient-care systems. For example, the da Vinci Surgical System, widely used in minimally invasive surgery, exemplifies embodied AI by enhancing surgeon precision, stability, and dexterity during procedures [21]. These systems often combine computer vision, sensor data, and real-time analytics to enable complex physical interactions, precise control, and increased safety during clinical procedures. Another critical area of embodied AI is robotic rehabilitation devices, which assist patients recovering from strokes, spinal cord injuries, or neurological conditions. These systems employ AI-driven feedback loops and adaptive algorithms to tailor therapy to individual patient needs, continually adjusting resistance, assistance, and motion pathways to optimize rehabilitation outcomes [10]. Embodied AI thus offers significant potential for enhancing clinical outcomes and patient safety, particularly in scenarios demanding high precision and personalized physical intervention.

While these systems operate in the physical realm, other forms of AI influence healthcare without a physical presence. Disembodied AI systems, in contrast, are software-based and do not have a physical presence. These include virtual clinical assistants, predictive analytic tools integrated within electronic health record (EHR) systems, and clinical decision-support tools. Disembodied AI systems leverage large-scale data analysis and machine learning algorithms to deliver diagnostic predictions, clinical insights, or personalized recommendations directly to clinicians through digital interfaces [3]. An example includes AI-driven predictive analytics embedded in EHRs that proactively identify patients at high risk of clinical deterioration, enabling timely medical intervention and potentially reducing adverse outcomes [20].

While embodied AI directly influences patient care through physical interaction, disembodied AI primarily enhances clinical decision-making and health management processes without direct physical patient interaction. Each approach offers unique benefits and challenges; embodied systems often raise safety and mechanical reliability concerns, while disembodied systems mainly contend with issues related to data privacy, transparency, and explainability [25].

Another frontier blurring the embodied/disembodied divide is wearable closed-loop drug-delivery. Smart insulin pumps use on-body sensors (continuous glucose monitors) plus embedded control algorithms to autonomously titrate insulin [5]. Although physically attached to the patient (embodied), their decision logic is cloud-updated and app-controlled (disembodied), illustrating how contemporary devices increasingly span both dimensions.

From Traditional Statistics to Machine Learning: Strengths, Limitations, and Transitions

Traditional statistical approaches in healthcare—such as linear and logistic regression, decision trees, and survival analysis—rely on explicit mathematical formulations to model relationships among variables within structured datasets. These methods often assume specific data distributions (e.g., normality or proportional hazards) and require predefined hypotheses, making them highly interpretable and transparent. Clinicians and researchers commonly use them for tasks such as risk prediction, outcome evaluation, and epidemiological modeling [11]. For example, logistic regression is frequently employed to predict binary outcomes such as disease onset, hospital readmission, or patient survival using predictors like age, comorbidities, or biomarker levels. Linear regression models are suited for continuous outcomes, such as blood pressure, while decision trees provide a rule-based framework for guiding referrals or testing based on symptoms or lab values. Survival models, such as Cox proportional hazards, are widely used to estimate time-to-event outcomes while accounting for censored data. These statistical models also play a foundational role in public health research—for example, in evaluating the effectiveness of vaccination programs, analyzing health disparities across populations, and forecasting disease burden. Their theoretical rigor and transparency make them well-suited for informing clinical guidelines, health policy, and regulatory decisions.

However, despite their strengths in interpretability and ease of implementation, traditional statistical methods face limitations when applied to high-dimensional, complex, or unstructured data types that are increasingly prevalent in modern healthcare. Examples include medical images, genomic sequences, free-text clinical notes, and electronic health records (EHRs). These data often violate key assumptions of classical models, such as linearity, independence, or normality, leading to reduced predictive accuracy and generalizability [3]. High-dimensional data can also result in overfitting or unstable parameter estimates, especially when the number of predictors exceeds the number of observations. Additionally, unstructured data—such as radiology reports or MRI images—cannot be easily reformatted into the structured, tabular inputs required by conventional statistical tools. These limitations are particularly pronounced in applications such as image classification, natural language processing (NLP), and modeling longitudinal disease trajectories. Traditional methods often struggle to capture nonlinear interactions, spatial or temporal dependencies, and latent features embedded in these datasets. As a result, there has been a shift toward more flexible, data-driven methods—especially machine learning (ML) and deep learning (DL)—which are better equipped to handle large, complex, and heterogeneous data sources.

While ML and DL are sometimes discussed together, they differ in important ways. Traditional ML models—such as random forests, support vector machines, and gradient boosting—are well-suited for detecting nonlinear relationships and handling mixed data types. These models generally require less computational power and smaller datasets compared to deep learning, making them more feasible for many real-world clinical tasks [14]. Deep learning, by contrast, involves multilayer neural networks capable of learning hierarchical feature representations from raw data. This architecture enables superior performance in tasks such as image classification and speech recognition, especially when dealing with large-scale, unstructured data. However, the trade-off is that DL models require significant computational resources (e.g., GPUs or cloud-based infrastructure) and large volumes of labeled data, which may be impractical in resource-constrained clinical settings.

The power of deep learning has been particularly evident in medical imaging. Convolutional neural networks (CNNs) (Fig. 2.2), a prominent class of DL models, have achieved human-level or superhuman performance in detecting pathologies like lung tumors in CT scans, breast cancer in mammograms, and diabetic retinopathy in retinal scans [6, 13]. Yet the complexity and opacity of these models pose challenges for interpretability and clinical trust, fueling interest in Explainable AI (XAI)—an emerging field aimed at making model decisions more transparent and clinically meaningful [1].

In conclusion, the shift from structured to complex and unstructured healthcare data has driven a transition from traditional statistical methods to more flexible, data-driven approaches like machine learning and deep learning. While classical

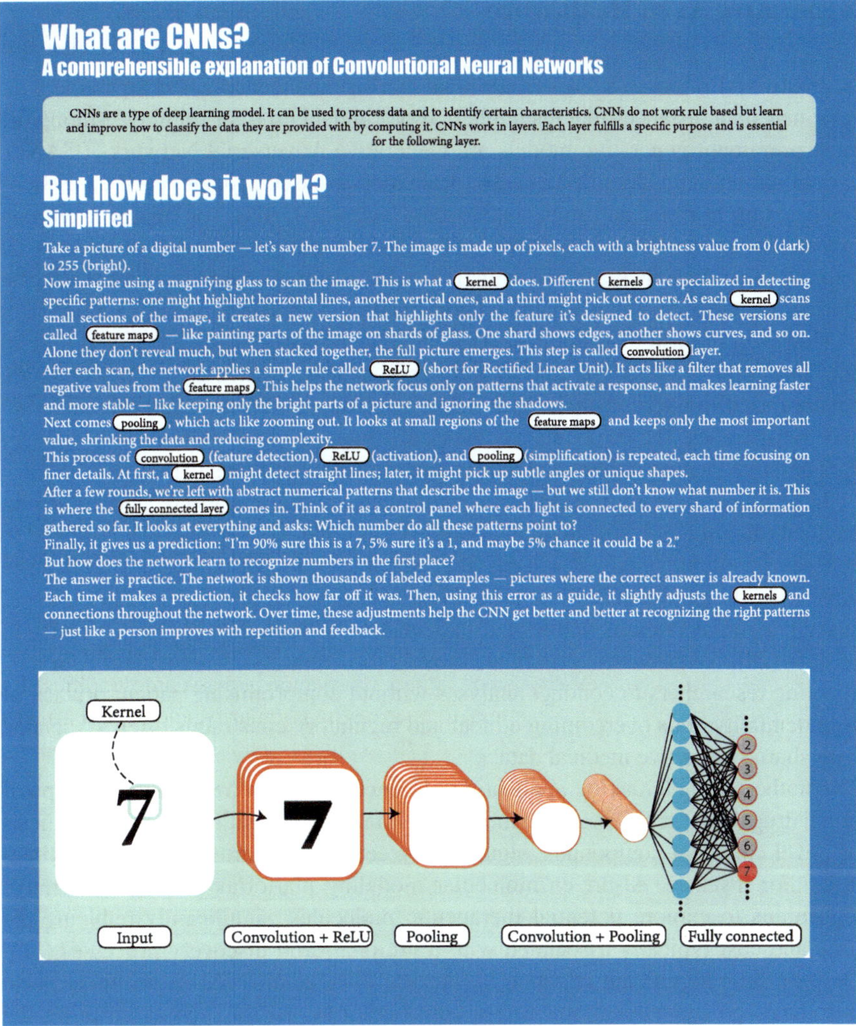

Fig. 2.2 What are convolutional neural networks? A short explanation

models remain valuable for their interpretability and transparency, they often encounter challenges and limitations when applied to modern data complexities. Machine learning addresses these challenges by capturing nonlinear patterns and accommodating diverse data types, while deep learning extends this capacity with powerful feature learning from raw inputs. Moving forward, blending statistical rigor with machine learning innovation offers a promising path—balancing accuracy, interpretability, and clinical feasibility.

Generative AI in Healthcare

Generative AI refers to a class of artificial intelligence techniques designed to generate new data instances that resemble real-world data used for training. Among the most prominent generative models are Generative Adversarial Networks (GANs), variational autoencoders (VAEs), and transformer-based models, each capable of synthesizing realistic and high-quality data outputs. GANs, for instance, employ two neural networks—a generator and a discriminator—engaged in adversarial training to produce increasingly realistic synthetic outputs, such as medical images, clinical scenarios, or textual data and conversations (chatbots such as ChatGPT).

However, the use of generative AI in healthcare raises critical concerns around data bias, ethical oversight, and model explainability, particularly when synthetic data are used in decision-making or diagnostic support. Without careful validation and transparency, these models risk perpetuating existing disparities in healthcare data and introducing unintended harms into clinical workflows [4].

In healthcare, generative AI has found meaningful applications, particularly in medical imaging and data augmentation. For example, GANs have been utilized to generate synthetic medical images that enhance training datasets, significantly improving the performance and robustness of diagnostic AI models. This is especially beneficial in cases where real patient data is limited, sensitive, or costly to acquire [28]. Additionally, generative models can create synthetic patient data sets, enabling researchers to conduct analyses without compromising patient privacy or confidentiality, thus overcoming ethical and regulatory constraints often associated with sharing sensitive medical data.

Another groundbreaking application of generative AI in healthcare is computational drug discovery. Generative models facilitate rapid identification and synthesis of novel chemical compounds, significantly accelerating drug development timelines. For instance, AI-driven molecular modeling platforms leverage generative algorithms to explore potential therapeutic molecules, significantly reducing the time and cost typically associated with traditional drug discovery processes [30]. Despite these significant advantages, the use of generative AI in healthcare also introduces critical ethical and safety considerations. Issues such as ensuring the quality of synthetic data and clinical validity, preventing biases from synthetic generation processes, and clearly delineating between real and generated patient data require careful management and rigorous oversight [25].

Regulators are taking notice. In 2023, the U.S. Food and Drug Administration (FDA) released draft guidance on the acceptable use of synthetic data to augment training and validation of medical-device algorithms, emphasizing provenance, fidelity testing, and disclosure requirements [8]. Such guidance signals a pathway for responsibly leveraging generative models while safeguarding patient safety and data integrity.

Data-Driven AI: Algorithms, Data, and Explainability

Data-driven healthcare AI typically employs tree ensembles, gradient boosting, support-vector machines, and—most prominently—deep neural networks for vision, language, and multimodal tasks. The performance of these systems is directly linked to the quality, volume, and diversity of training data, making data curation and preprocessing essential to reduce bias and improve generalizability [3]. High-quality, representative data are prerequisites. Common pitfalls include missingness, measurement error, and sampling bias [20].

Explainability and transparency in data-driven AI systems—called Explainable AI (XAI)—are critical to fostering clinician trust, improving patient safety, and ensuring regulatory compliance. XAI techniques, such as Local Interpretable Model-agnostic Explanations (LIME) and SHapley Additive exPlanations (SHAP), have gained prominence in healthcare as tools for elucidating AI decision-making processes [1]. While useful, these approaches often fall short in complex clinical workflows or treatment planning scenarios.

Recent research has advanced the field by exploring task- and action-level explanations. For example, Michalowski et al. [17, 18] developed an explainability component within an AI-driven system called MitPlan, designed to manage multimorbid patients. Their approach goes beyond traditional model explainability by offering "Level 3" explanations that clarify why a clinical action was chosen, why modifications were made, and how factors such as cost or patient adherence influenced those choices. The authors demonstrated that such structured, multi-aspect explanations significantly improved physicians' understanding of the treatment plan rationale and enhanced trust in the system's recommendations [17]. This work has major ramifications for care interventions for addition healthcare providers including nursing.

Building on this, an exploratory study evaluated the use of large language models (LLMs) like Meditron70B to automatically generate treatment explanations. The study found that LLM-generated explanations can complement or even match the quality of manually curated ones, particularly in dimensions like evidence reflection and self-containment. However, the researchers also cautioned against potential "hallucinations" and clinical inaccuracies that require validation and oversight [18]. This highlights the potential and limitations of generative AI tools in high-stakes clinical environments as well as health professional training environments.

Together, these studies illustrate a growing consensus: explainability must be actionable, clinically relevant, and context-aware, especially in domains like multimorbidity, where decision support systems must reconcile overlapping and sometimes conflicting guidelines. Approaches combining automated planning, structured medical and health knowledge, and advanced NLP models pave the way toward more interpretable and trustworthy AI in healthcare. Data quality is paramount for successful AI deployment in healthcare. Poor data quality, including missing data, measurement errors, biased datasets, or lack of representativeness, can significantly compromise algorithm performance and lead to incorrect conclusions or harmful patient outcomes [20]. Consequently, rigorous data preprocessing and validation processes are essential to ensure data reliability, reduce biases, and improve the generalizability of AI models. Data harmonization, privacy-preserving techniques, and standardized data protocols also facilitate integrating and effectively utilizing data from diverse healthcare settings.

Given the implications for patient safety, regulatory bodies such as the FDA increasingly emphasize explainability and transparency as critical factors when evaluating AI-based medical devices and software tools [9]. As AI continues to integrate into healthcare practice, the ongoing development and refinement of explainability methods will be necessary to bridge the gap between AI capability and clinical acceptance.

Ethical Considerations and Human Oversight

Integrating artificial intelligence into healthcare presents significant ethical challenges that must be addressed proactively. Chief among these concerns are patient privacy and data protection, especially given the sensitivity of healthcare information. With AI systems often requiring extensive patient data, there is an inherent risk of privacy breaches, unauthorized data sharing, or misuse of sensitive information [25]. Ensuring robust data governance frameworks, secure data handling practices, and clear informed consent processes are essential to mitigate these risks and maintain patient trust.

Bias in AI algorithms represents another substantial ethical challenge. Algorithms trained on biased datasets may reinforce or amplify existing healthcare disparities, leading to unfair treatment or differential access to care among certain populations [19]. For example, AI-driven predictive algorithms have been shown to exhibit biases that systematically disadvantage racial or socioeconomic groups if training data reflect existing inequalities or insufficient diversity. Addressing algorithmic bias involves rigorous testing, continuous monitoring, and inclusive data collection practices to ensure equitable outcomes across all patient groups [20].

Accountability and transparency in AI decision-making processes are critical ethical considerations. Clinicians and healthcare organizations must clearly understand how AI tools reach specific clinical decisions to maintain accountability, properly explain to patients, and ensure compliance with legal and ethical standards [1]. The increasing complexity of AI models, particularly deep learning, complicates transparency and makes interpretability a key ethical and practical requirement. Beyond national guidelines, the European Union AI Act [7] classifies most medical AI as "high-risk," mandating rigorous quality-management systems, post-market monitoring, and transparency artefacts. Such supranational legislation will likely influence global best practice and harmonization efforts.

Finally, the central role of human oversight cannot be understated. While AI offers powerful tools for enhancing clinical capabilities and decision-making, the ultimate responsibility for patient care must remain with healthcare professionals.

Maintaining human oversight involves delineating the roles and responsibilities of clinicians, providing appropriate AI training and education, and ensuring continuous human involvement in validating, interpreting, and applying AI-generated insights in clinical settings [23]. Human oversight safeguards against potential AI-related errors, biases, or ethical missteps, reinforcing the responsible integration of AI into healthcare practice. Moreover, human engagement in all aspects of AI development, testing, and by implementation ensure preservation and advancement of what it means to be human.

Illustrative Case Studies in Healthcare

Case Study 1: Radiology Imaging

Radiology has significantly benefited from the integration of AI, particularly deep learning algorithms. Convolutional neural networks (CNNs), specifically designed for image recognition and analysis, have consistently demonstrated the capability to match or surpass radiologists' performance in identifying abnormalities in medical images. For instance, CNN-based AI tools have achieved remarkable accuracy in detecting breast cancer lesions from mammograms, often identifying subtle features that human experts might overlook [16]. Similar successes have been noted in detecting lung nodules, identifying early signs of stroke on brain imaging, and accurately classifying various dermatological conditions from skin images [6].

Such AI-driven diagnostic tools significantly enhance radiologists' efficiency by automating routine image analyses, providing preliminary diagnostic interpretations, and prioritizing urgent cases. This allows radiologists to focus their expertise on complex or ambiguous cases, ultimately improving diagnostic accuracy and patient outcomes. Importantly, these tools are designed to augment, not replace, radiologists—providing second opinions or highlighting regions of interest for closer review. However, ensuring AI systems integrate smoothly into clinical workflows, maintaining transparent decision-making processes, and addressing potential biases from training datasets remain ongoing challenges for broader adoption [1]. Interpretability tools, such as saliency maps, help radiologists visualize which image features influenced the AI's prediction, enhancing trust and clinical validation.

Key takeaway Deep-learning–based triage systems can improve diagnostic accuracy and radiologist efficiency, but their clinical value depends on proper bias mitigation, explainability, and calibration of model confidence to avoid overreliance in ambiguous cases.

Case Study 2: Patient Monitoring and Predictive Analytics

AI-driven predictive analytics embedded within electronic health record (EHR) systems have become increasingly important for early identification of patient deterioration, improving patient and hospital safety, and reducing preventable harm. Algorithms leveraging data such as vital signs, laboratory results, clinical notes, and historical patient information can predict adverse events, including sepsis, cardiac arrest, or hospital readmissions, well before traditional clinical warning signs manifest [20].

For example, hospitals implementing AI-driven early warning systems have significantly reduced adverse clinical events, as clinicians receive timely alerts prompting early intervention and preventive measures. These predictive tools exemplify disembodied AI—operating as virtual clinical assistants that enable proactive rather than reactive care delivery [3]. These systems function passively in the background, continuously analyzing patient data without user interaction and surfacing only when predefined clinical thresholds are met.

Key takeaway AI-powered early warning systems can transform clinical care from reactive to proactive, but their success hinges on reducing false positives, integrating into workflows, and maintaining clinician trust.

Case Study 3: Personalized Medicine

AI has also profoundly impacted personalized medicine, particularly through advances in genomic analysis and individualized treatment planning. Machine learning models analyzing genomic data can accurately predict individual responses to therapies, identify genetic predispositions for specific diseases, and tailor therapeutic interventions precisely to a patient's genetic makeup [2]. For instance, AI models have been used to predict response to trastuzumab in HER2-positive breast cancer [6] or to flag CYP2C19 variants that influence response to clopidogrel [3].

In oncology, AI-driven genomic analyses facilitate targeted therapy selection based on tumor-specific mutations, significantly improving therapeutic efficacy and reducing adverse effects compared to traditional one-size-fits-all approaches [6]. Furthermore, pharmacogenomic applications of AI can predict adverse drug reactions and optimize medication choices and dosages based on individual genetic profiles, thus enhancing patient safety and treatment outcomes [2]. While personalized medicine leveraging AI promises significant improvements in healthcare delivery, addressing ethical concerns around genetic data privacy, equitable access to genomic testing, and the interpretation of complex genomic information remains essential for its successful implementation [25]. This includes establishing robust consent frameworks for the secondary use of genomic data in research or commercial development.

Key takeaway Genomic machine learning enables precision therapy tailored to individual biology, but its full impact depends on equitable access to sequencing and transparent consent for secondary data use.

Outlook and Conclusions

Integrating Artificial Intelligence (AI) and Big Data into healthcare has initiated a paradigm shift in how medical and health information are analyzed, interpreted, and acted upon. As demonstrated through multiple use cases—from radiology imaging and predictive patient monitoring to personalized genomic medicine—AI technologies have already begun to enhance clinical workflows, diagnostic accuracy, and treatment personalization. These advancements are primarily attributed to data-driven methodologies, including deep learning and generative models, which have shown exceptional capabilities in analyzing complex, high-volume, and high-dimensional healthcare data [6, 29].

However, this rapid evolution presents significant challenges. Ethical concerns surrounding data privacy, algorithmic bias, transparency, and informed consent remain at the forefront. The opaque nature of many AI algorithms, especially deep learning systems, has triggered ongoing discourse on explainability, accountability, and the need for robust human oversight in clinical decision-making [1, 25]. Ensuring that AI systems do not unintentionally exacerbate health disparities or erode patient trust is critical to their safe and equitable implementation.

Looking ahead, the future of AI in healthcare will be defined not just by technological advancement but by the human relationships and effectiveness of interdisciplinary collaboration across healthcare providers, data scientists, ethicists, and policymakers. Regulatory frameworks must evolve with technology to support transparency, ensure safety, and maintain fairness. Education and training will also equip clinicians with the knowledge and confidence to work alongside AI tools, interpret their outputs, and retain final responsibility for patient care.

As AI systems become increasingly embedded in the clinical environment, ongoing research will be necessary to validate their effectiveness in diverse populations and care settings. Additionally, advances in explainable AI (XAI), federated learning (which allows AI models to be trained without centralized data sharing), and privacy-preserving analytics will help mitigate many current limitations and ethical concerns. Ultimately, the promise of AI in healthcare can only be realized through conscientious, transparent, and human-centered whole person integration that prioritizes patient, family and community well-being above all.

In the near term, multimodal foundation models that fuse imaging, text, waveforms, and genomics (e.g., GPT-4-based Med-PaLM Multimodal) promise unified reasoning across disparate data sources. Success will hinge on federated-learning protocols, synthetic-data safeguards, and transparent evaluation benchmarks that reflect real-world diversity.

Useful Resources

Beam AL, Kohane IS. Big data and machine learning in health care. JAMA. 2018;319:1317–8. https://doi.org/10.1001/jama.2017.18391.

Esteva A, Robicquet A, Ramsundar B, Kuleshov V, DePristo M, Chou K, et al. A guide to deep learning in healthcare. Nat Med. 2019;25:24–9. https://doi.org/10.1038/s41591-018-0316-z.

Topol EJ. Deep medicine: how artificial intelligence can make healthcare human again. Basic Books; 2019.

Review Questions

Here are some examples:

1. What distinguishes rule-based from data-driven AI?
2. How do embodied AI systems differ from disembodied AI?
3. Why is deep learning particularly suitable for medical image analysis?
4. Discuss the role of generative AI in healthcare.
5. What ethical considerations must be addressed when implementing AI in healthcare?

Answers to Review Questions

1. Rule-based AI applies explicit, predefined rules, whereas data-driven AI learns from data without explicit instructions.
2. Embodied AI involves physical interactions (e.g., robots), whereas disembodied AI involves software-based virtual interactions.
3. Deep learning excels in recognizing complex patterns within unstructured data, such as medical images, improving diagnostic accuracy.
4. Generative AI can create synthetic medical data, improve training scenarios, and expedite drug discovery.
5. Ethical considerations include privacy protection, minimizing bias, maintaining transparency, and ensuring accountability.

References

1. Amann J, Blasimme A, Vayena E, Frey D, Madai VI. Explainability for artificial intelligence in healthcare: a multidisciplinary perspective. BMC Med Inform Decis Mak. 2020;20:310.
2. Ashley EA. Towards precision medicine. Nat Rev Genet. 2016;17:507–22.
3. Beam AL, Kohane IS. Big data and machine learning in health care. JAMA. 2018;319:1317–8.
4. Chen IY, Szolovits P, Ghassemi M. Can AI help reduce disparities in general medical and mental health care? AMA J Ethics. 2021;23:E121–7.
5. Dadlani V, Pinsker JE, Dassau E, Kudva YC. Advances in closed-loop insulin delivery systems in patients with type 1 diabetes. Curr Diab Rep. 2018;18:88.
6. Esteva A, Robicquet A, Ramsundar B, Kuleshov V, DePristo M, Chou K, et al. A guide to deep learning in healthcare. Nat Med. 2019;25:24–9.
7. European Parliament & Council. Regulation (EU) 2024/… on harmonised rules for artificial intelligence (AI Act). Brussels: Author; 2024.
8. Food and Drug Administration. Artificial intelligence-enabled device software functions. 2023. https://www.fda.gov/medical-devices/medical-device-regulatory-science-research-programs-conducted-osel/addressing-limitations-medical-data-ai.

9. Food and Drug Administration. Artificial intelligence-enabled device software functions: lifecycle management and marketing submission recommendations. 2025. https://www.fda.gov/media/184856/download.
10. Gassert R, Dietz V. Rehabilitation robots for the treatment of sensorimotor deficits: a neurophysiological perspective. J Neuroeng Rehabil. 2018;15:46.
11. Harrell FE. Regression modeling strategies. 2nd ed. Cham: Springer; 2015.
12. Henry KE, Hogan CA, Gafni A, Ramamoorthy V, D'Costa S, Sorkin JD, et al. A targeted realtime early warning score (TREWScore) for septic shock. Sci Transl Med. 2015;7:299ra122.
13. Litjens G, Kooi T, Bejnordi BE, Setio AA, Ciompi F, Ghafoorian M, et al. A survey on deep learning in medical image analysis. Med Image Anal. 2017;42:60–88.
14. Lucas PJF, van der Gaag LC, Abreu G. Bayesian networks in biomedicine and health-care. Artif Intell Med. 2004;30:201–14.
15. Maddox TM, Embí P, Gerhart J, Goldsack J, Parikh RB, Sarich TC. Generative AI in medicine – evaluating progress and challenges. N Engl J Med. 2025;392:2479–83. https://doi.org/10.1056/NEJMsb2503956.
16. McKinney SM, Sieniek M, Godbole V, Godwin J, Antropova N, Ashrafian H, et al. International evaluation of an AI system for breast cancer screening. Nature. 2020;577:89–94.
17. Michalowski M, Wilk S, Michalowski W, Rao M, Carrier M. Provision and evaluation of explanations within an automated planning-based approach to solving the multimorbidity problem. J Biomed Inform. 2024;156:104681.
18. Michalowski M, Wilk S, Bauer JM, Carrier M, Delluc A, Le Gal G, et al. Manually curated versus LLM-generated explanations for complex patient cases: an exploratory study with physicians. In: Cornet A, Martin-Sánchez F, editors. Artificial intelligence in medicine: proceedings of AIME 2024. Cham: Springer; 2024. p. 333–43.
19. Obermeyer Z, Powers B, Vogeli C, Mullainathan S. Dissecting racial bias in an algorithm used to manage the health of populations. Science. 2019;366:447–53.
20. Rajkomar A, Dean J, Kohane I. Machine learning in medicine. N Engl J Med. 2019;380:1347–58.
21. Rivero-Moreno Y, Echevarria S, Vidal-Valderrama C, Pianetti L, Cordova-Guilarte J, Navarro-Gonzalez J, Acevedo-Rodríguez J, Dorado-Avila G, Osorio-Romero L, Chavez-Campos C, Acero-Alvarracín K. Robotic surgery: a comprehensive review of the literature and current trends. Cureus. 2023;15:e42370.
22. Shortliffe EH, Buchanan BG. A model of inexact reasoning in medicine. Math Biosci. 1975;23:351–79.
23. Topol EJ. Deep medicine: how artificial intelligence can make healthcare human again. New York: Basic Books; 2019.
24. Vaswani A, Shazeer N, Parmar N, Uszkoreit J, Jones L, Gomez AN, Kaiser Ł, Polosukhin I. Attention is all you need. In: Advances in neural information processing systems. Curran Associates, Inc. 2017;30(NIPS 2017):5998–6008.
25. Vayena E, Blasimme A, Cohen IG. Machine learning in medicine: addressing ethical challenges. PLoS Med. 2018;15:e1002689.
26. Wang Y, Wang L, Rastegar-Mojarad M, Moon S, Shen F, Afzal N, et al. Clinical information extraction applications: a literature review. J Biomed Inform. 2018;77:34–49.
27. Weng W-H, Wagholikar KB, McCray AT, Szolovits P, Chueh HC. Medical subdomain classification of clinical notes using a machine learning-based natural language processing approach. BMC Med Inform Decis Mak. 2017;17:155.
28. Yi X, Walia E, Babyn P. Generative adversarial network in medical imaging: a review. Med Image Anal. 2019;58:101552.
29. Yu KH, Beam AL, Kohane IS. Artificial intelligence in healthcare. Nature Biomed Eng. 2018;2:719–31.
30. Zhavoronkov A, Ivanenkov YA, Aliper A, et al. Deep learning enables rapid identification of potent DDR1 kinase inhibitors. Nat Biotechnol. 2019;37:1038–40.

Chapter 3
Human Intelligence and the Caring Imperative

Ursula H. Hübner

Learning Objectives
- To understand the principles of human decision making while relying on rational and non-rational agents
- To understand how evidence-based medicine and nursing shape decision making
- To understand social and emotional intelligence and its impact on caring
- To understand the models of the patient-provider relationship
- To analyze how AI can alter the patient-provider relationship

Key Terms
- Human Decision-Making Theories
- Evidence Based Medicine and Nursing
- Social Intelligence
- Emotional Intelligence
- Patient-provider relationship
- Patient-provider-technology relationship

Summary
This chapter expands on the concept of human intelligence as introduced in Chap. 1. It lays the foundation of understanding decision making, a major expression of human intelligence. Decision making might only be governed by the rational deliberation of the utility of an outcome, but research has shown that non-rational components may also strongly influence decision making. We, therefore, give a short account of utility theory, prospect theory and regret theory. In medicine and nursing, evidence-based practice offers a methodology to strengthen the rational basis of decision making through evidence from studies while also respecting the values and preferences of patients. To better understand the breadth of human intelligence, we

U. H. Hübner (✉)
School of Business Management and Social Sciences,
Osnabrück University of Applied Sciences, Osnabrück, Germany

U. H. Hübner et al. (eds.), *Bridging Artificial and Human Intelligence*, Health Informatics, https://doi.org/10.1007/978-3-032-11938-4_3

provide an introduction to social and emotional intelligence while highlighting their influence on improving care and contributing to the provider-patient relationship. Different types of provider-patient relationships are presented while emphasizing the role of narrative medicine when developing an empathetic relationship. When introducing technology—in particular AI—the dyadic relationship emerges as a triad in which AI may affect the provider, the patient, and their interaction. Considering medicine and healthcare as both science and art, AI should harness the scientific side rather than the art side. While AI models excelled in performing individual isolated tasks, AI tools could not match human experts when complex, real world tasks in patient care had to be mastered. Although AI technology is intriguing and promises technical innovation in care, it is the well-being of the patients that remains at the core of medicine, nursing, and healthcare.

Human Decision-Making in Medicine and Healthcare

Principles of Human Decision

In Chap. 1, we introduced the concept of human intelligence and its various aspects. Decision-making is considered a key feature that hallmarks human intelligence. Before addressing decision-making in the context of medicine, we will begin with a brief overview of decision-making in general with a focus on economics since that is where it is a widely discussed topic.

Expected utility theory, as one of the most influential theories in economics, posits that decisions are made through purely rational deliberation, aiming to maximize the expected utility of the outcome. This theory dominated economic discussions for a long time until it was challenged by alternative theories, such as prospect theory. Prospect theory, grounded in observations of actual human behavior, suggests that people tend to avoid losses in risky decisions since losses are perceived as having more significant consequences than equivalent gains. According to prospect theory, there are two types of behavior: *risk aversion* in case of gains and *risk seeking* in case of losses. When an outcome is framed as a gain, individuals tend to prefer a highly certain outcome with lower utility over a less certain outcome with higher utility (risk aversion). Conversely, when faced with potential losses, individuals often prefer an uncertain – but potentially high – loss over a certain but smaller loss, anticipating that the uncertain event may not occur [1]. The following situations A and B illustrate the behavior of risk aversion and risk seeking with an example from a lottery.

A - **Gain scenario: 100% to win 500 points (preferred)** versus 50% to win 1000 points and 50% to win 0 points

B - **Loss scenarion:** 100% to lose 500 points versus **50% to lose 1000 points and 50% to lose 0 points (preferred)**

This framing—whether an outcome is viewed as a gain or a loss—significantly influences decision-making behavior [1]. Developed by the psychologists Kahneman and Tversky, prospect theory is based on experiments in cognitive psychology and introduces the concept of decision-making under uncertainty. They argue that human judgment is governed by heuristics, which simplify complex facts, along with their related subjective probabilities and values. These heuristics are employed in various situations, such as

- determining the probability of whether an event belongs to a specific class based on **stereotype** information or
- based on the **frequency or size** of this class and thereby the availability of the information, and
- predicting numerical values based on the **reference points** or anchors previously given.

While these heuristics can be useful in making quick judgments, they can also lead to significant biases that may even influence experts in a field [2].

In risky situations, human decision-making is influenced by additional biases. For instance, past decisions can shape future choices as individuals strive for consistency. Moreover, readily accessible and easily recalled options are often favored over those requiring more effort to gather information, such as seeking out reviews or statistics. The idea that biases can influence our decisions suggests that choices are frequently not made through deliberate, rational, and conscious processes, but are instead largely governed by the unconscious [3].

Today, many scientists concur regarding the existence of two types or systems of decision-making. The first system operates quickly, relying on automatic, unconscious processes, while the second system is slower, involving effortful, intentional, and conscious thought. It is suggested that only the second type, or system II, accesses the capacity-limited working memory, accounting for its slower operation. When comparing expert and novice decision-making, experts typically reach conclusions quickly and intuitively, whereas novices require more time to analytically arrive at a decision. However, experts relying on intuition may encounter challenges when faced with novel situations that necessitate the adaptation of their fast, unconscious processes [4].

Translating These Principles into Healthcare

Prospect theory has also been applied to healthcare, as decisions made by healthcare providers and patients alike often involve risks, with potential gains such as the benefits of healthy behavior or improved quality of life, and potential losses such as the harms of unhealthy behavior or reduced life expectancy. Many studies in healthcare have focused on the effect of framing in various scenarios, such as promoting healthy habits like physical activity, healthy eating, sun protection, and smoking cessation. This has been well illustrated in a bibliometric study and scoping review

[5]. The review also highlighted that framing was examined in studies on its impact on anti-COVID-19 measures, such as physical distancing and vaccination. The outcome of both of those are associated with high uncertainty. With a loss-aversion mindset, individuals tended to accept these measures more readily when the messaging emphasized avoiding losses, rather than acquiring gains [5].

Another decision-making theory applied to healthcare is regret theory. This theory suggests that decisions are based not only on utility appraisal but also on the anticipation of feelings of regret or rejoicing when comparing the outcomes of alternative choices. In healthcare, regret may arise from, for example, omitting a diagnostic test that could have provided crucial information for treatment. Similar to prospect theory, regret theory belongs to a group of approaches that consider non-rational factors influencing decision-making, specifically the emotions of regret and rejoicing [6].

In the context of the dual system model, which differentiates between fast, affective, unconscious thinking (system I) and slow, intentional, conscious thinking (system II), regret has been incorporated into a decision model as a proxy for system I, while utility considerations represent system II. This decision model explained the behavior of physicians who only treated patients with a very high probability of developing a pulmonary embolism, which was likely due to the anticipated regret of causing bleeding through anticoagulant therapy. If only rational arguments were considered, patients with much lower probabilities would also have been treated, as system II would evaluate the net benefits/harms ratio of the drugs and would arrive at this decision. The interaction between system I and system II thinking can lead to both undertreatment and overtreatment of patients [7].

Evidence Based Practice: A Healthcare Model for Decision-Making

In medicine and nursing, evidence-based practice aims to provide the best possible rational basis (evidence) for decision-making, while also incorporating personal experience. In addition to relying on evidence, this approach advocates decisions that consider patient values and preferences.

The increasing number of randomized controlled trials (RCTs) and systematic reviews has paved the way for evidence-based medicine. This movement has been bolstered by healthcare providers' growing awareness of the importance of accessing the most recent and comprehensive findings to effectively treat their patients. Evidence-based medicine relies on data used in epidemiological and biostatistical analyses of patient and population studies, contrasting with earlier approaches that prioritized habit and tradition. Through meta-analyses, it aims to synthesize all of the available findings to offer decision aids, such as odds ratios, which can be integrated into clinical judgments. This approach has driven lifelong learning in medicine and was instrumental in establishing the Cochrane Collaboration. As care increasingly involves interdisciplinary and interprofessional teams, evidence-based practice provides a common foundation for communication, decision-making, and the sharing of responsibilities [8].

With the explosion in the number of studies being published, the need for systematic summaries of the most recent and robust evidence is more urgent than ever. This urgency introduces increased pressure to promptly provide such summaries after study findings are released. Although the imperative to produce up-to-date practice guidelines, including recommendations and clinical algorithms, is longstanding, progress has been impeded by the inherent limitations of human research teams, e.g., in terms of time and financial resources. Efforts to automate the creation of evidence summaries are also not new [9], but recent advances using large language models have accelerated these efforts. While tests of these models for tasks such as information retrieval (e.g., PICO extraction), synthesis of RCTs, and simplifying medical texts for dissemination purposes indicate considerable potential, they also reveal limitations in factual consistency and domain accuracy. Therefore, current findings still underscore the need for rigorous human expert oversight [10].

Further Concepts of Human Intelligence

We have learned herein above that decision-making, as a core aspect of intelligent human behavior, is governed by both rational and non-rational factors. In healthcare, evidence-based practice adopts a normative approach, outlining how patient care should be conducted. This approach aims to expand the factual basis for clinical judgments by incorporating both experience and patient preferences. In the first chapter, we established the understanding that human intelligence is not a singular concept but rather allows for multiple perspectives. In patient-centered healthcare, the focus extends beyond managing diseases to addressing individuals who are dealing with these conditions. This approach leverages the patient-provider relationship to facilitate health improvement and healing as well as stabilization and palliation. Recognizing humans as social beings who lead successful lives largely due to their social skills and emotional capacities, the constructs of social and emotional intelligence have emerged. Although they are interrelated, these constructs have developed along different paths and, therefore, need to be presented separately.

Originating in the 1920s and 1930s, social intelligence was initially defined as the "ability to understand and manage people" [11]. Today, it is recognized as distinct from academic intelligence and comprises social understanding, social memory, and social knowledge, making it a multi-trait concept [12]. This definition aligns with cognitive concepts of intelligence, but it specifically focuses on understanding, storing, and retrieving social stimuli and their contexts, such as faces, names, and both verbal and non-verbal communication.

In contrast, emotional intelligence primarily pertains to the individual rather than a group. It also utilizes cognitive abilities and is defined as the "ability to reason about and use emotions to enhance thought". Building on this concept, emotional intelligence involves the capacity to perceive, monitor, discriminate, and manage one's own and others' emotions to achieve the desired goals [13].

Both social and emotional intelligence, particularly the latter, have been utilized to enhance the understanding of clinicians' behavior and performance. Research has shown that problem-solving skills in nurses are influenced not only by perceived academic achievement and solution-focused thinking but also by emotional intelligence [14]. Similarly, it has been demonstrated that emotional intelligence can improve the work performance of nurses. In this context, emotional intelligence was divided into the components of well-being, self-control, emotionality, and sociability. Well-being and sociability were found to enhance both task performance and contextual performance, while self-control positively affected task performance alone. In addition, both emotionality and sociability were associated with a reduction in counterproductive work behaviors [15]. Similar effects resulted from a path-analysis study on physicians (Fig. 3.1), revealing that the emotional intelligence of physicians and the rate of patient follow-up visits positively influenced patient trust. The patient-physician relationship effectively mediated the translation of patient trust into patient satisfaction and directly enhanced patient satisfaction [16]. This study underscores the intricate network of positive effects on patient satisfaction shaped by emotional intelligence.

In addition to medical knowledge, social intelligence, personal characteristics, and organizational acumen are integral components of clinical competencies. These elements have been identified as training goals for preparing interns for their workplace and clinical duties [17]. This perspective supports the idea that individuals can be trained to achieve these goals, aligning with the concept that emotional intelligence is more of a developable state than an innate trait. Indeed, training measures such as social perspective taking have been shown to improve emotional intelligence over time. However, these improvements do not occur immediately but

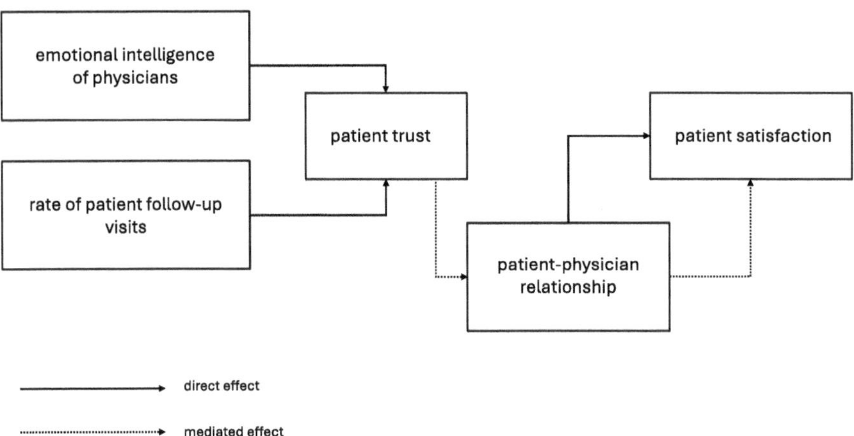

Fig. 3.1 Mediating role of the patient-provider relationship

typically manifest after about six months, suggesting the need for ongoing practice to allow these skills to mature [18].

The question of whether emotional intelligence is uniquely human or can be approximated by machines is intriguing. In an experiment on video-based reasoning involving emotional intelligence, questions about scenes were presented to both humans and a large language model (LLM) for analysis. Humans and the LLM exhibited distinct response patterns. Humans utilized non-verbal information and considered context, the temporal dynamics of the scene, and the cultural background. They also acknowledged when questions could not be answered. In contrast, the LLM was more cautious with insufficient information, relying on specific utterances and interpreting scenes literally. However, it was adept at identifying the tone, atmosphere, and central figures of the scene. The study's authors suggest these findings indicate a promising potential for advancing LLMs in digital applications requiring social intelligence [19]. In a similar study, an LLM demonstrated the ability to identify and describe emotions from a scene report, performing above the population norm in an Emotional Awareness test. This capability is being considered for use in an LLM-based training tool for mental health patients with emotional awareness impairments, helping them develop skills for perceiving and describing emotions [20]. These examples present realistic use cases and applications in specific areas. However, whether these capabilities align with the broader concept of human emotional intelligence remains uncertain.

The Patient-Provider Technology Relationship

Human intelligence, as a cognitive resource for reasoning, forms the foundation of the patient-provider relationship. This encompasses not only human intelligence in general but also its specialized forms, such as social and emotional intelligence. As aforementioned, emotional intelligence plays a critical role in developing trust among patients, which is then translated into satisfaction through the patient-physician relationship [16].

As a complex and multifaceted agent, the patient-physician relationship can manifest in various gestalts. According to the four classical models proposed by Emanuel and Emanuel, this relationship can be described as

1. paternalistic,
2. informative,
3. interpretative, and
4. deliberative.

In the paternalistic model, the physician acts as the patients guardian, making decisions on their behalf according to objective criteria. This approach aims to maximize patient well-being, often at the expense of patient autonomy. The informative model regards the patient-physician relationship as an engineering model, where the physician provides the scientific information that the patient lacks. Armed with these facts, the patients then make decisions based on their own values. The interpretative model views the relationship as a means to uncover the patient's values, which may be obscured. Here, the physician's role is to provide necessary information to help elucidate these values. Finally, the deliberative model positions the physician as someone who suggests values within the context of the diagnosis and available treatment options. The patient and physician then deliberate on these values together to reach a decision [21].

Although Emanuel and Emanuel only refer to the physician, the four models can be easily transferred to nurses and other healthcare professionals. In modern medicine and nursing, the paternalistic model is generally considered the least appropriate form of interaction between patients and healthcare professionals, except in cases where the patient explicitly requests that the provider act on their behalf. This model can undermine patient autonomy and does not address the current focus on patient-centered care, which values shared decision-making and respects the patient's preferences and values.

Both the interpretative and deliberative models emphasize the importance of healthcare providers listening to and valuing patients' narratives. This aligns with narrative medicine, which is a formal approach that harnesses patients' stories for diagnostic and treatment purposes. Narrative medicine draws on cognitive, symbolic, and affective means to interpret the meaning and significance within these stories. For patients, sharing their illness narrative can be a therapeutic act, while for physicians and nurses, it serves as a rich source of information. This information can evoke memories, associations, and allusions, thereby unlocking creative potential for both diagnostic and therapeutic interventions. Through a collaborative process, providers and patients work together to uncover the meaning behind signs, symptoms, and values [22].

Compassion is another component of the patient-provider relationship. It describes the "[…] attitude of active regard for another's welfare with an imaginative awareness and emotional response […]" [23]. Family physicians and community nurses are particularly well-positioned to develop long-term patient-provider relationships, which can include a strong component of compassion. As Uygur and colleagues argue, compassion may develop when it is considered a core value that motivates providers to behave compassionately. It further requires the necessary energy and capacity, and it is stimulated through connections such as the possibility to develop a sustained patient-physician relationship [23].

This dyadic relationship transforms into a triad with the introduction of technology, particularly AI, as a third partner. AI can influence the relationship through the provider or the patient individually, but it also has the potential to affect the overall dynamic of the relationship itself.

AI Affecting the Provider

From the perspective of physicians, AI can serve as a tool, assistant, or peer [24]. These roles can significantly influence how AI impacts the patient-provider relationship. When AI acts as a peer, it likely has the greatest influence on the provider. In such cases, it is crucial for the provider to make the role of AI transparent to the patient. This includes explaining how the provider and the AI system work together as well as clarifying the reasons for adopting or not adopting the AI system's recommendations.

The discussion surrounding who benefits most from AI system support is ongoing and controversial. Some studies suggest that young providers and novices gain as AI helps them develop skills and solve specific problems. Conversely, other research indicates that more experienced practitioners can better evaluate, appraise, and utilize the AI system's output. Therefore, tailoring AI support to different expertise levels is advisable, challenging the notion that a universal approach works for everyone. In addition, it is argued that AI-assisted decision-making fundamentally differs from traditional methods, necessitating relearning and practical experience [24].

Another way that AI can impact providers is through an intrinsic tendency to favor machine-generated decisions over human ones, including their own, which is known as automation bias [25]. Research has shown that less qualified and less adept diagnosticians are more prone to this bias, often accepting incorrect AI recommendations more readily than their more skilled colleagues [26]. Moreover, further findings highlight that correct AI support is the most powerful driver for enhancing human diagnostic accuracy. Likewise, incorrect AI support can significantly impair diagnostic judgment. Although diagnostic performance, previous training, and working experience were also found to positively influence the diagnostic result, their impact was less effective than that of the AI model [27].

AI Affecting the Patient

The availability of health information on the Internet has shown the potential to enhance the health literacy of people. Similarly, the use of educational material incorporated in health apps can contribute to changing the lifestyle toward healthier behavior and a higher awareness for healthy living. Along this path, the use of AI tools—particularly large language models—is the next step as a door opener for having even more information at your fingertips. In addition, AI tools may be instrumental not only for accessing more information but for summarizing the information found in diverse sources on the Web. However, all of the promises have fallen short when the information is presented in a way that is not suitable for non-experts, misleading, or even incorrect. In the past, various measures were taken to ensure the credibility of the information on the Web and in apps [28]. However, there is the need for a new approach to this problem in light of the enhanced expressiveness of AI tools. With the help of large language models, information can be presented in a way that meets the patient's needs and level of understanding, thereby allowing for tailored information. However, the linguistic fluency and proficiency of large language models can also instill confidence and trust in spurious information. Particularly LLM enabled chatbots employed for patient counselling can be a double-edged sword. While available 24 h and 7 days/week, which is helpful for patients in need, they might also act as trusted partners building an illusion of unjustified reality. Given the circumstance that LLMs can fabricate facts, they might contrive "patient stories" and simply make up lies. This might become dangerous in situations when vulnerable patients, for instance persons suffering from cancer, are seeking help [29]. Overseeing chatbots and other AI tools to be used by patients and consumers in general becomes imperative. AI knowledgeable healthcare providers can guide their patients to make use of the right tools in the right situation.

AI and Technology Shaping the Patient-Provider Relationship

When debating how AI and technology may alter patient-provider interactions, it is important to bear in mind that medicine and healthcare are both art and science. As Saunders noted, the art of medicine incorporates rules of thumb that go beyond objective scientific knowledge. Good doctors often resort to the art of medicine to validate their judgments. Similarly, it should be remembered that "Doctors treat patients, not X-rays. Such treatment is both a science and an art" [30]. This raises the question of whether AI can shape only the scientific aspect or also the art component. This is particularly relevant in situations when patients and healthcare professionals are establishing their relationship.

Patient involvement and respect for patient preferences are core values of person-centered care and can lead to shared decision-making. This patient-oriented mindset contrasts with the paternalistic model of care, allowing for richer interactions between patients and providers. However, there is concern that AI could dictate treatments without considering patient priorities or acknowledging value-plurality. Such a development might revert to old paternalistic practices, affecting both patients and providers by undermining their autonomy, i.e., the autonomy of the providers to make use of their competencies and the autonomy of the patients to stick to their own values [31].

It is promised that AI could serve as a time saver for physicians, freeing them to engage in empathetic relationships with their patients. However, even if these time savings are realized, there is no guarantee that this extra time will be used to improve the patient-provider relationships. On the contrary, some argue that more time does not necessarily translate into the time needed to practice empathy [32]. Instead, it may be redirected to increase patient throughput, especially when seen from an organizational standpoint.

In the provider-patient-AI triangle, AI is required to prove its trustworthiness either through reliability (explainability and validity) or through a high level of accuracy and certainty. It is argued that, in the absence of explainability, the use of AI tools could still be morally justified when they are highly efficient and enhance health benefits due to their accuracy. Similarly, other complex medical devices, such as those used in medical imaging, typically do not provide explanations of how they compute the images. Despite this lack of explainability, healthcare providers consider these tools valuable due to the precise insights they offer into body structures and functions. Ultimately, AI becomes a meaningful tool in the provider-patient relationship if it contributes to preserving a good human-to-human empathetic relationship and respects the autonomy of the providers and patients. In other words, AI should not interfere with practicing medicine and healthcare as an art [33].

When AI "Outperforms" Humans ...

There is a plethora of studies demonstrating the excellent performance of AI systems in individual tasks, sometimes even outperforming senior healthcare providers and experts. This has been shown, among others, in a study where even a clinically less demanding diagnostic task was mastered more accurately by an AI model than by clinicians with no pertinent formal qualification [34]. Furthermore, AI systems outperformed clinical experts in medical tasks that were more challenging, such as the medical licensing exam [35]. Comparing human and AI performance raises not only the question about the best AI systems but also about who the best performing humans are. While a pertinent formal qualification and training is an undebated prerequisite to work accurately other factors such as work experience and job title may play a minor or no role at all. Clinical expertise was found to comprise a formal qualification and training in the field and by a high level of self-confidence in one's own clinical capacity. These findings underscore the fact that not only the clinical academic background, but also psychological characteristics contribute to developing a high degree of expertise [34].

However, when inspecting the literature of human vs. AI performance in healthcare, most studies rely on a single specialized task paradigm often involving diagnostic skills. When testing the performance for a complex combination of clinical tasks that resemble real world scenarios, different results emerged. Such a combination was realized in a study that investigated the human and AI abilities of an autonomous decision-making task comprising information-gathering, adherence to the guidelines and instructions as well as robustness to information order and information quantity. Medical doctors achieved significantly higher accuracy values in three out of the four conditions tested. It was only for the most simple to diagnose condition (appendicitis) that LLMs and humans performed equally well. None of the LLMs could provide clinically meaningful recommendations for the required combination of treatments. The accuracy of LLMs did not increase when more information was made available, which points out the LLMs' deficiency in selecting and focusing on essential information. Furthermore, if the order of information changed, then the accuracy of the diagnostic performance of LLMs changed as well [35]. It could be argued that it is only a matter of time until LLMs are trained well enough to exhibit the same capabilities as humans. Therefore, further investigations are deemed necessary.

Other studies point to AI as a tool for enhancing the clinical capacity of healthcare providers. This perspective seems more realistic and promising than merely looking at the competition between AI and humans. Many researchers and professional bodies, therefore, call for AI literacy among healthcare providers and the necessary educational measures. Proficiency in incorporating AI output in the clinical workflow and tasks would help providers optimize the benefits offered by AI and minimize the risks entailed by AI. We have expanded on what the didactic goals and approaches could look like in Chap. 1. Medical and Nursing Schools are responsible for adopting new basic courses or blending AI knowledge with the content of the existing traditional courses to ensure up-to-date academic education in this field. It is also the obligation of professional associations to offer continuing education in AI particularly as the field is evolving and new challenges will be emerging. The caring imperative should guide the course development and its implementation.

Conclusions and Outlook: The Caring Imperative

Human decision-making is a complex process that is subject to non-rational and rational forces. This fact is reflected by the concept of system I and system II thinking, the fast intuitive vs. the slower deliberative way of reaching decisions. The interaction of both systems plays an important role in daily life but it is also affecting professional decision-making. Particularly in healthcare, there are circumstances where humans can capitalize on the way these systems work. Whereas the fast thinking mode is required in emergency cases, the slower mode is advantageous in complex treatment planning for example. Although evidence-based practice aims at fostering the scientific and thereby rational basis of decision making, it also gives room for personal experience and patients' subjective values. Providing care by humans for humans further depends on social and emotional intelligence as a resource for managing people and for using emotions to enhance thought. The patient-provider relationship is a good example of where these competencies can be leveraged to support the process of obtaining good health outcomes. With the advent and increasing use of AI tools, this relationship is exposed to changes. It can be altered through affecting the provider and the patient individually or the relationship as such. These changes may encompass both benefits and risks. Although there are instances where AI systems outperform human experts, particularly in solving isolated tasks, human experts possess the singular capability of providing care in an authentic and holistic manner. This does not preclude the use of AI tools. Therefore, health professionals must be well equipped and prepared for these new challenges while following the caring imperative.

Useful Resources

Patient-Provider Relationship: 5 Principles. https://www.techtarget.com/patientengagement/news/366584767/5-Principles-to-Build-Positive-Patient-Provider-Relationships

Developing Relationships. https://link.springer.com/chapter/10.1007/978-3-030-29271-3_3

Review Questions

1. What are the core statements of utility theory, prospect theory, and regret theory?
2. Please give some examples of their application in healthcare.
3. What are the aims of evidence-based practice and how can AI support the generation of evidence?
4. Please give some examples of how social and emotional intelligence can influence the provision of care.
5. Please describe the different models of the patient-provider relationship.
6. How can AI influence the patient-provider relationship?

Answers to Review Questions

1. Utility theory posits that decisions are made on utility evaluation seeking to maximize its utility. Prospect theory suggests that decisions depend on whether the outcome is framed as a gain or loss and that people are avoiding losses because they loom larger than gains. In regret theory, decisions are governed by the anticipation of feelings of regret or rejoicing when comparing the outcomes of alternative choices.
2. Following the assumptions of utility theory, clinicians would base their decision on the benefit-harm ratio of a drug and choose the prescription of the drug if this ratio exceeds a certain threshold. In prospect theory, people would accept measures, e.g., COVID-19 containment measures, if they contributed to avoiding losses rather than obtaining gains. In regret theory, a diagnostic decision about ordering a test would be determined by whether you would regret not having ordered it.
3. Evidence-based practice aims at providing the best possible overview and summary of the most recent, high-quality studies on which clinicians can base the care for their patients. It also incorporates personal experience and advocates for respecting patient values and preferences. AI can support this process in many ways, for example through supporting the process of summarizing studies and hereby contributing to the collection and appraisal of findings.
4. Social intelligence and emotional intelligence help providers shape the patient-provider relationship, help elicit treatment priorities from patients, and then discuss them in a meaningful and goal-directed manner.

5. Following Emanuel and Emanuel, there are four models of a patient-provider relationship, i.e., the paternalistic, informative, interpretative, and deliberative model. They differ along a continuum with regard to respecting, eliciting, discussing, and developing patient values and preferences. They also differ regarding the role and obligations of the healthcare providers who are either a guardian, engineer, consultant, or friend.
6. AI can affect the provider, patient, or the entire relationship. Providers should be aware of the pitfall that they might too readily accept the recommendations of the AI system without questioning the output. They should also make sure that the role of AI is explained properly to the patient. This does not necessarily mean that they have to explain the functioning of the algorithms, but rather the accuracy, reliability, and validity of the recommendation. Patients can be affected when using chatbots to obtain help or advice. They should be aware that chatbots, which can feign an atmosphere of understanding and compassion, are machines and there is an illusion surrounding them. Finally, the relationship can be affected if the autonomy of the patient and the provider are at stake. This might happen when the AI system dictates recommendations and thereby imposes a paternalistic style. All of these risks can be avoided if providers manage AI in a responsible way, educate their patients, and double-check the output of the system.

References

1. Kahneman D, Tversky A. Prospect theory: an analysis of decision under risk. Econometrica. 1979;47:263–91. https://doi.org/10.2307/1914185.
2. Tversky A, Kahneman D. judgment under uncertainty: heuristics and biases. Science. 1974;185:1124–31.
3. Johnson J. Chapter 12 – Human decision-making is rarely rational. In: Johnson J, editor. Designing with the mind in mind. 3rd ed. Morgan Kaufmann; 2021. p. 203–23. https://doi.org/10.1016/B978-0-12-818202-4.00012-X.
4. Evans JS. Dual-processing accounts of reasoning, judgment, and social cognition. Annu Rev Psychol. 2008;59:255–78. https://doi.org/10.1146/annurev.psych.59.103006.093629. PMID: 18154502
5. Gisbert-Pérez J, Martí-Vilar M, González-Sala F. Prospect theory: a bibliometric and systematic review in the categories of psychology in web of science. Healthcare (Basel). 2022;10:2098. https://doi.org/10.3390/healthcare10102098.
6. Loomes G, Sugden R. Regret theory: an alternative theory of rational choice under uncertainty. Econ J. 1982;92:805–24.
7. Djulbegovic B, Hozo I, Beckstead J, Tsalatsanis A, Pauker SG. Dual processing model of medical decision-making. BMC Med Inform Decis Mak. 2012;12:94. https://doi.org/10.1186/1472-6947-12-94.
8. Sackett DL, Rosenberg WM. The need for evidence-based medicine. J R Soc Med. 1995;88:620–4. https://doi.org/10.1177/014107689508801105.
9. Djulbegovic B, Guyatt GH. Progress in evidence-based medicine: a quarter century on. Lancet. 2017;390:415–23. https://doi.org/10.1016/S0140-6736(16)31592-6.

10. Li J, Deng Y, Sun Q, Zhu J, Tian Y, Li J, Zhu T. Benchmarking large language models in evidence-based medicine. IEEE J Biomed Health Inform. 2024;29:6143–56. https://doi.org/10.1109/JBHI.2024.3483816.
11. Thorndike RL, Stein S. An evaluation of the attempts to measure social intelligence. Psychol Bull. 1937;34:275–85. https://doi.org/10.1037/h0053850.
12. Weis S, Süß H-M. Reviving the search for social intelligence – a multitrait-multimethod study of its structure and construct validity. Personal Individ Differ. 2007;42:3–14. https://doi.org/10.1016/j.paid.2006.04.027.
13. Mayer JD, Salovey P, Caruso DR. Emotional intelligence: new ability or eclectic traits? Am Psychol. 2008;63:503–17. https://doi.org/10.1037/0003-066X.63.6.503. PMID: 18793038.
14. Selçuk Tosun A, Akgül Gündoğdu N, Avci D, Gündüz ES. Determinants of problem-solving skills of nursing students: solution-focused thinking skills and emotional intelligence. J Eval Clin Pract. 2025;31:e14312. https://doi.org/10.1111/jep.14312.
15. Galanis P, Katsiroumpa A, Moisoglou I, Derizioti K, Gallos P, Kalogeropoulou M, Papanikolaou V. Emotional intelligence as critical competence in nurses' work performance: a cross-sectional study. Healthcare (Basel). 2024;12:1936. https://doi.org/10.3390/healthcare12191936.
16. Weng HC. Does the physician's emotional intelligence matter? Impacts of the physician's emotional intelligence on the trust, patient-physician relationship, and satisfaction. Health Care Manag Rev. 2008;33:280–8. https://doi.org/10.1097/01.HCM.0000318765.52148.b3.
17. De Villiers M, Van Heerden B, Van Schalkwyk S. 'Going the extra mile': Supervisors' perspectives on what makes a 'good' intern. S Afr Med J. 2018;108:852–7. https://doi.org/10.7196/SAMJ.2018.v108i10.13052.
18. Gorgas DL, Greenberger S, Bahner DP, Way DP. Teaching emotional intelligence: a control group study of a brief educational intervention for emergency medicine residents. West J Emerg Med. 2015;16:899–906. https://doi.org/10.5811/westjem.2015.8.27304.
19. Mori E, Qiu Y, Kataoka H, Aoki Y. A comprehensive analysis of a social intelligence dataset and response tendencies between Large Language Models (LLMs) and humans. Sensors (Basel). 2025;25:477. https://doi.org/10.3390/s25020477.
20. Elyoseph Z, Hadar-Shoval D, Asraf K, Lvovsky M. ChatGPT outperforms humans in emotional awareness evaluations. Front Psychol. 2023;14:1199058. https://doi.org/10.3389/fpsyg.2023.1199058.
21. Emanuel EJ, Emanuel LL. Four models of the physician-patient relationship. JAMA. 1992;267:2221–6.
22. Charon R. Narrative medicine: a model for empathy, reflection, profession, and trust. JAMA. 2001;286:1897–902. https://doi.org/10.1001/jama.286.15.1897. https://jamanetwork.com/journals/jama/fullarticle/194300.
23. Uygur J, Brown JB, Herbert C. Understanding compassion in family medicine: a qualitative study. Br J Gen Pract. 2019;69(680):e208–16. https://doi.org/10.3399/bjgp19X701285.
24. Göndöcs D, Dörfler V. AI in medical diagnosis: AI prediction & human judgment. Artif Intell Med. 2024;149:102769. https://doi.org/10.1016/j.artmed.2024.102769. Epub 2024 Jan 20. PMID: 38462271.
25. Goddard K, Roudsari A, Wyatt JC. Automation bias: a systematic review of frequency, effect mediators, and mitigators. J Am Med Inform Assoc. 2012;19:121–7. https://doi.org/10.1136/amiajnl-2011-000089.
26. Kücking F, Hübner U, Przysucha M, Hannemann N, Kutza JO, Moelleken M, Erfurt-Berge C, Dissemond J, Babitsch B, Busch D. Automation bias in AI-decision support: results from an Empirical Study. Stud Health Technol Inform. 2024;30(317):298–304. https://doi.org/10.3233/SHTI240871.
27. Kücking F, Busch DA, Przysucha M, Kutza JO, Hannemann N, Hüsers J, Babitsch B, Hübner U. Impact of AI recommendation correctness on diagnostic accuracy in clinical decision-making. Int J Med Inform. 2025;13(207):106223. https://doi.org/10.1016/j.ijmedinf.2025.106223.

28. Boyer C. Quality and safety of health mobile applications: are they an issue? In: Hübner UH, Wilson GM, Shaw Morawski T, Ball MJ, editors. Nursing informatics: a health informatics, interprofessional and global perspective. Cham: Springer; 2022.
29. Lawson McLean A, Hristidis V. Evidence-based analysis of AI chatbots in oncology patient education: implications for trust, perceived realness, and misinformation management. J Cancer Educ. 2025;40:482–9. https://doi.org/10.1007/s13187-025-02592-4.
30. Saunders J. The practice of clinical medicine as an art and as a science. West J Med. 2001;174:137–41.
31. Lorenzini G, Arbelaez Ossa L, Shaw DM, Elger BS. Artificial intelligence and the doctor-patient relationship expanding the paradigm of shared decision making. Bioethics. 2023;37:424–9. https://doi.org/10.1111/bioe.13158.
32. Rubeis G. Ethics of medical AI. Cham: Springer; 2024.
33. Sauerbrei A, Kerasidou A, Lucivero F, Hallowell N. The impact of artificial intelligence on the person-centred, doctor-patient relationship: some problems and solutions. BMC Med Inform Decis Mak. 2023;23:73. https://doi.org/10.1186/s12911-023-02162-y.
34. Kücking F, Hübner UH, Busch D. Diagnostic accuracy differences in detecting maceration between humans and artificial intelligence: the role of human expertise revisited. JAMIA. 2025;32:1425–33.
35. Hager P, Jungmann F, Holland R, Bhagat K, Hubrecht I, Knauer M, Vielhauer J, Makowski M, Braren R, Kaissis G, Rueckert D. Evaluation and mitigation of the limitations of large language models in clinical decision-making. Nat Med. 2024;30:2613–22. https://doi.org/10.1038/s41591-024-03097-1. Epub 2024 Jul 4. PMID: 38965432; PMCID: PMC11405275.

Part II
Innovation and AI Strategies

Chapter 4
Leadership for Innovation in AI

Angela Barron McBride

Learning Objectives
- Define leadership so it encompasses what the healthcare professional does in seeking IT/AI solutions to problems
- Develop a sense of IT/AI developmental tasks in five career stages for both healthcare clinicians and educators
- Increase understanding of how important the change process is to innovation

Key Terms
- Leadership
- Career stages
- Innovation
- The change process
- Challenges for AI-assisted decision making

Summary
This chapter defines leadership, so it encompasses what the non-specialist does in steering novel IT/AI solutions to challenges and problems. IT/AI developmental tasks are outlined for five career stages, bearing in mind some differences between clinicians and educators. Innovation and leadership are concepts that have much in common because both are concerned with inspiring and catalyzing others to achieve institutional mission by designing new ways of achieving long-held values. The imperative for leadership is to drive organizational innovation by fostering an environment that embraces and encourages the use of technology, including AI. Steps in the change process are discussed: establishing a need for the proposed change; assembling the group who will lead the effort; developing and communicating the

A. B. McBride (✉)
Indiana University, Bloomington, IN, USA
e-mail: ambride@iu.edu

U. H. Hübner et al. (eds.), *Bridging Artificial and Human Intelligence*, Health Informatics, https://doi.org/10.1007/978-3-032-11938-4_4

plan; encouraging new behaviors and risk taking; communicating with stakeholders; implementing and evaluating changes made; hardwiring new systems; and celebrating successes.

Introduction

Healthcare educators and clinicians are regularly urged to exert leadership and be innovative, but what those admonitions entail is not always clear. If anything, one sometimes has the impression that saying it often enough, particularly in a world that increasingly values solutions to problems that involve information technology (IT) and augmented intelligence (AI), is thought to be the key to leadership and innovation happening. Reality is much more complex. Experienced healthcare professionals dominate formal leadership positions—C suite, directors, deans, managers, committee chairs—and they may downplay the importance of IT/AI strategies because they did not come of age professionally in a time full of helpful apps much less the expectation of leveraging advancements in computing and data to move care forward. Even those generations of healthcare professionals who grew up familiar with simulation learning and knowing how to use the electronic health record (EHR) to monitor patterns of behavior may think that using AI-related approaches in practice, education and research is the responsibility only of those with graduate degrees in healthcare informatics and not their responsibility because they have graduate degrees in medicine, nursing, pharmacy, physical therapy and the like. But that is not the case.

It is healthcare leaders who are not experts in IT/AI who are most likely to have to decide whether innovative technologic solutions to healthcare problems are going to be developed, implemented, evaluated, and sustained. That is why today's healthcare leaders must be prepared to consider IT/AI-informed possibilities as part of their career development and understand enough about the change process so they can oversee the needed innovations in practice, education and/or research. There is an urgency to healthcare professionals exerting such leadership as exemplified in President Biden's farewell address on January 15, 2025, when he warned about the "profound possibilities and risks" that come with artificial intelligence [1].

The principal undertaking of leadership is inspiring and catalyzing others to achieve institutional mission and shared goals in circumstances where the context—e.g., reimbursement policies, financial situation, regulatory environment, clinical expectations, perceptions of health and aging, workforce availability—is evolving, thus the ongoing need to design new ways of achieving long-held values [2]. Values do not change but contexts do for every generation of healthcare providers. That definition of leadership incorporates the three major views of leadership that have surfaced in the last century: (a) leadership as personal—the ability to inspire and catalyze others; (b) leadership as achieving institutional mission—effectively meeting goals and wished-for outcomes; and (c) leadership as getting ready for tomorrow—innovatively addressing challenges resulting from an evolving context. This definition of leadership is useful—from fledgling clinician to award-winning healthcare educator—because leadership is not envisioned as a matter of administrative title, but a complex skill set exercised in service to purpose by all licensed healthcare professionals and one that may regularly involve IT/AI strategies. This view of leadership includes individual performance and productive teamwork, plus inspiring higher performance in others, and hopefully the eventual creation of enduring excellence. This viewpoint embraces not only what healthcare professionals do personally but what they accomplish through others.

Benner's From Novice to Expert was one of the first writings to make clear that there is a journey all healthcare professionals undertake in life after licensure as they move from novice to competent then proficient on the way to expert [3]. The advantage of a framework with multiple stages is that professionals do not expect to be fully developed at the beginning of their careers, and that approach can be particularly useful in conceptualizing how healthcare leaders who are not specialists in informatics might be involved in developing, implementing, evaluating and sustaining AI solutions over the course of their careers. It is the non-specialist leaders who are most likely to play the biggest role in steering the change process necessary for successful innovation.

Career Stages

Table 4.1 outlines developmental tasks to be accomplished in five career stages noting some differences between the tasks to be accomplished by the clinical leader as opposed to the academic leader. This approach builds on Dalton, Thompson and Price's classic article on stages of a professional career [4]. Stages are a heuristic device for describing key transitions in focus over the course of a career, but reality is often messy, and a person can be in one stage but already involved in some of the activities of other stages. The main advantage of a stage model is that it helps professionals focus on what is developmentally appropriate for where they are and not expect to be fully developed at the start of a career, and it provides a road map for where they are going career-wise.

The first career stage is **Preparation**. The central activity is learning, and the primary relationship is as a student. The major theme of this stage is assimilating the values, knowledge base, clinical and inquiry skills important to one's healthcare profession and the overall field of health care. Formal education—undergraduate, graduate, postgraduate—is the best way to master a body of knowledge, but you also need a variety of socialization experiences—mentoring, clinical rotations, internships, assistantships, residencies, workshops, conferences, etc.—to hone your problem-solving skills and develop competencies that complement formal course work. A class might include accessing and using evidence-based information, but an internship might require computer competencies that you learn on your own or develop via resources available in the practice setting. In a real way, formal

Table 4.1 Developmental tasks by career trajectory

Stage	Master clinician	Faculty member

Preparation	• Formal education—undergraduate, graduate
	  o Learn IT/AI basics, e.g., information literacy, computer competencies, use of information management systems, data analysis, accessing and using evidence-based information, using data for research and development, using virtual assistants, cybersecurity
	• Internships, apprenticeships, workshops
	• Licensure/Certification
	• Join appropriate professional organizations
		• Formal education—undergraduate, graduate, post-doctoral research training
		  o Learn IT/AI basics, e.g., information literacy, computer competencies, use of information management systems, data analysis, accessing and using evidence-based information, using data for research and development, using virtual assistants, cybersecurity
		• Internships, apprenticeships, workshops
		• Licensure/Certification
		• Experience as teaching assistant and/or research assistant
		• Mentored presentations, publications, small grants
		• Join appropriate professional organizations

Independent contributions	• Ensure that personal practice reflects best practices and outcomes set by organization
	• Build teamwork
	  o Get to know IT/AI expertise within organization, learn how to hire such expertise for your team
	• Participate in governance structure where professional standards are developed
	  o Raise possibilities of AI-enhanced care
	  o Suggest need for additional cybersecurity policies
	• Preceptor students
	  o Learn from them new developments in IT/AI
	• Demonstrate emotional intelligence
		• Build research team and program of scholarship—interdisciplinary connections, refereed presentations and publications, external funding
		  o Get to know IT/AI expertise within organization, learn how to hire such expertise for your team and how to build virtual teams
		• Integrate teaching, research, and service commitments
		  o Investigate the use of AI-powered simulation to enhance clinical decision-making skills
		  o Suggest need for additional cybersecurity policies
		• Advise/mentor students
		  o Learn from them new developments in IT/AI
		• Demonstrate emotional intelligence
		• Develop reputation in area of excellence

(continued)

Table 4.1 (continued)

Stage	Master clinician	Faculty member

Development of home setting	• Engage in strategic planning
	  ○ Build the culture of innovation
	• Lead quality-improvement efforts
	  ○ Provide support and resources for AI adoption
	• Juggle multiple responsibilities
	• Develop junior colleagues
	• Build home setting's image (presentations/publications), infrastructure, and resources
	• Obtain additional preparation for leadership
	• Demonstrate diversity intelligence
	  ○ Mindful of algorithm bias in AI
	• Represent organization elsewhere
		• Engage in strategic planning
		  ○ Build the culture of innovation
		• Lead curricular and program initiatives
		  ○ Provide support and resources for AI adoption
		• Juggle multiple grants/projects
		• Develop junior colleagues
		• Build home setting's image, infrastructure, and resources
		• Obtain additional preparation for leadership
		• Extend own program of scholarship
		• Consider policy and product consequences of own research
		• Demonstrate diversity intelligence
		  ○ Mindful of algorithm bias in AI
		• Represent organization elsewhere

Development of field/health care	• Consult in area of expertise
	• Serve as advisor to local, regional, national, and/or international efforts and organizations
	• Assume leadership roles in professional organizations
	  ○ Build programs and resources for continuous AI learning
	  ○ Reward innovation
	• Develop next generation of leaders
	  ○ Encourage spirit of innovation
	• Speak out about issues of the day locally, regionally, and nationally
	• Testify regarding needed policy changes, e.g., legal, ethical and safety guidelines for AI in health care
		• Consult in area of expertise
		• Serve as advisor to local, regional, national, and/or international efforts and organizations
		• Assume leadership roles in professional organizations
		  ○ Build programs and resources for continuous AI learning
		  ○ Reward innovation
		• Develop next generation of leaders
		  ○ Encourage spirit of innovation
		• Write integrative papers geared toward summarizing what is known and not yet known
		• Testify regarding needed policy changes, e.g., legal, ethical and safety guidelines for AI in health care

The gadfly (wise person) period	• Take on special assignments
	• Serve as a consultant
	• Coach current leaders
	  ○ Encourage innovation using AI
	• Push dialogue and challenge new ways of thinking
		• Take on special assignments
		• Serve as a consultant
		• Coach current leaders
		  ○ Encourage innovation using AI
		• Push dialogue and challenge new ways of thinking

A version of this table first appeared in Chapter 5 of McBride's [2, pp. 67–68]

education helps you "read the lines" and socialization experiences help you "read between the lines," and both are important in orchestrating a career.

So important is informatics to the education of healthcare professionals that technologic requirements for professional accreditation now exist. For example, undergraduate nursing programs increasingly include coursework covering basic computer skills, EHR usage, data analysis, healthcare technology applications, patient data management, and the ability to use information systems to improve patient care. Students are expected to apply these skills in real-world settings. A framework of globally-accepted core competencies in health informatics has been developed for nursing that can prepare fledgling leaders who are open to IT/AI-enhanced innovations [5]. Since technology keeps changing, the authors of that framework note that what constitutes core competencies here and now will continue to change over time, so technology-related preparation is appropriately reframed to include the essential concept of continuous learning as one moves to other career stages.

The Accreditation Council for Graduate Medical Education has also developed *Clinical Informatics Milestones* that track informatics abilities from Level 1 to Level 5 with the expectation of moving from novice to expert resident or fellow in a specialty or subspecialty [6]. The behavioral milestones are designed for developmental purposes to support continuous quality improvement, so are in keeping with this career-stage model. One milestone bearing on consumer informatics applications moves from discussing a health informatics application (Level 1) to leading implementation of a novel consumer-focusing health informatics application. That is a good example of the kind of journey a non-informatics specialist might undergo, first learning about existing consumer-focused health informatics applications then eventually steering the change process necessary to develop and test new applications at a later stage.

Once you learn IT/AI basics, you are hopefully sensitized to the fact that technology-related learning is all around, so you go to conferences and workshops paying attention to how AI was incorporated into clinical decision making, an educational experience, or a research protocol. You may decide to be on the lookout for how membership in a professional organization can help you keep current about existing AI applications in your specialty area. Not only is it important to master agreed-upon basics in this career stage, but it is important to realize how essential ongoing familiarity with IT/AI applications will be to health care in the twenty-first century even if you do not aspire to become an expert in this area.

The second career stage, **Independent Contributions**, focuses on moving from fledgling abilities to competence, and operating as a collegial professional. The major theme of this stage is dealing with the inevitable gap between ideals learned and the realities of the work setting. Whether you are a clinician or an educator, this is a time for developing your nascent skills further, learning to do high-level juggling, figuring out the strengths of the organization so that you can take advantage of them, working with students, getting to know the expertise within the organization and team building. Many of these developmental tasks involve some aspects of IT/AI. Thinking about how to improve your practice or your program of scholarship raises questions about whether there might be AI-assisted solutions to difficulties. Getting to know the IT/AI expertise within the organization can be useful to your team building, and it can also lead you to think beyond your organization's strengths to the possibilities offered by virtual teams and learning how to maximize their effectiveness. As you get to know informatics specialists within your organization, you learn more about options and how to ask questions, so you can take advantage of their services and are in a better position to hire additional expertise in that area. Precepting or teaching students forces the educator to keep up with new developments, though younger learners are often likely to be more knowledgeable about assistive technologies and social communication than their teachers, thus the real opportunity for teachers to also learn new things from their students.

If you are a clinician involved in the governance structure of your facility, your knowledge of IT/AI basics may lead you to ask questions about whether the institution's cybersecurity policies are adequate, a questioning that may lead the organization's IT experts to get more involved in the concerns of your setting. If you are an educator, you may realize that your school is not doing a very good job inculcating the IT/AI basics into the curriculum, so you sign up to work on the committee concerned with remedying this situation. What knowledge of the basics does for you at this stage is open your thinking up to new possibilities.

The better you get as a clinician or educator, the more you think about how difficulties or challenges might be more effectively addressed. It is wanting to improve matters that usually propels healthcare professionals to the next career stage, **Development of the Home Setting**. This is a time when the focus switches from being primarily concerned about personal development to assuming more responsibility for organizational development and the enhancement of others, perhaps serving as a Committee Chair or holding some formal administrative position. The theme of this stage is building the home setting's image, infrastructure and resources, and in the process moving personally from competence to added expertise. This is a time for managing multiple projects, strategic planning, developing and leading new initiatives, and building a culture of innovation and collaboration. The more you seek to improve the organization, the more you find yourself involved in quality-improvement efforts, cost containment and redesigning systems, all of which may require support and resources for AI adoption. Since the focus is on the organization, the professional at this career stage must also be aware that systems being proposed may have been developed with limited input from some patient populations thus there might be algorithm bias that needs to be addressed. It is in trying to change the organization that you often become more familiar with the legal, ethical and cybersecurity issues involved in encouraging AI innovation.

This is the career stage when you are most likely to learn more about the change process—how do you get buy-in and take advantage of the enthusiasm of "early adopters," how do you get new resources and where do you get them from, who are the stakeholders that need to be part of any solution and what's the best way to communicate with them, can we say that the change has been reliably delivered over time, what are reasonable outcomes, do we have systems in place to collect needed data, what do we do to institutionalize new practices and systems, how do we build morale and risk taking, how do we use any successes in service to the next level of development. Even if you have not had any formal education in administration, getting involved in developing the home setting forces the individual to think long and hard about the change process, and to learn from successes, mistakes and false starts.

The more you are involved in the development of your own organization, the more you are likely to take an active role in **Development of the Field/Health**

Care, the fourth career stage. Now you become more invested in shaping the overall future of your profession and health care, more often serving on an advisory board and acting as a consultant. The theme of this period is using your hard-won authority to create a better tomorrow. Asked to assume a leadership role in some professional organization, you become involved in promoting the profession's image, infrastructure and resources or in lobbying for policy changes needed or best practices that will improve care giving. Seeking to upgrade practice at this level may lead you to urge that a new office or committee be constituted to help others figure out whether AI can be useful to them. The American Psychological Association's Office of Health Care Innovation did just that in creating a "Companion Checklist: Evaluation of an AI-Enabled Clinical or Administrative Tool" which serves as a guide for psychologists considering the integration of clinical tools utilizing artificial intelligence into their practice [7]. Leadership at this career stage might also involve persuading the national or international organization for which you have assumed a governance role to establish new annual awards that recognize pioneering breakthroughs in care delivery models or educational interventions using AI, thus encouraging further innovation in this area.

When you hold a leadership position in either a discipline-specific organization (e.g., American Academy of Nursing) or an interdisciplinary organization (e.g., Gerontological Society of America), there is ample opportunity to raise new issues about how AI is shaping best practices and what safeguards need to be in place. Though a number of professional associations have developed position papers on the use of artificial intelligence in practice, there still are many organizations oblivious to the ethical issues—lack of transparency, privacy and accountability, bias and discrimination, safety and security problems, the potential for criminal and malicious use—that have been identified by informatics specialists but which remain undiscussed in groups whose members do not have that background but need that information [8]. This lack provides the nonspecialist leader with an opportunity to raise awareness and help the organization better address the challenges members face.

The fifth career stage, **The Gadfly (Wise Person) Period**, is when you are in your so-called retirement or "preferment" years and continue to be generative when no longer constrained by institutional obligations. You continue to shape the field as a coach, board member or consultant. At this stage professionals are very experienced, but no longer inhibited as they once were, by having to represent their work settings so they can now speak freely about their personal beliefs. This is a time when many retirees take on special assignments, connect across sectors, and push dialogue. They may be asked to coach some of today's leaders who are seeking to introduce AI innovations. Having had a full career, the retiree can be frank and push the dialogue, so others recognize there are many pathways to "solutions." Even though you were never an expert in informatics, individuals in that specialty might even ask you to write a Foreword to a book that they are writing about IT/AI innovations because you are known to have encouraged innovation along the way. If you decide at this stage to reflect on the leadership you have exerted in the field, you might choose to write up a case study critically describing the AI-assisted advances you facilitated.

What is clear is that no healthcare provider or educator who functions in a leadership role can avoid being involved with IT/AI-assisted protocols and practices at any stage of development now and in the coming decades. ChatGPT, DeepSeek and similar programs are fast becoming work staples. Smart wearables for patient monitoring are getting more and more effective and expanding what it means for caregivers to encourage self-help. Digitally augmented cognitive technology is making mental health therapy available to patients who cannot access an in-person therapist. Large scale analytics are increasingly helpful in uncovering patterns of behavior, leading to more timely interventions when there's complexity and rarity involved. In this rapidly changing environment, leadership involves helping others tolerate ambiguity, deal with technologic overload, select the appropriate tools, manage connectivity, lead virtual teams and encourage a lifelong-learning approach to digital skills. It is not possible to list how IT/AI will color every developmental task over the course of a career; what is important is to realize that learning the basics early on will hopefully strengthen your leadership capabilities because otherwise you could not ask relevant questions. IT/AI applications offer great potential to make health care better, but that potential will only be realized if caregivers nurture innovation and understand how to manage the change process.

Innovation and the Change Process

Innovation is the process of bringing about new approaches, processes, services, solutions, products or devices that have a significant positive effect on existing challenges. Innovation and leadership are concepts that have much in common because both are concerned with inspiring and catalyzing others to achieve institutional mission by designing new ways of achieving long-held values and goals. In today's AI world, healthcare leaders must be prepared to manage innovation no matter their specialty or setting. Leaders do not need to be technologic experts themselves, but they must understand the change process enough to appreciate the difference between knowing what to do and getting it done. Too often experts think they know what to do, but they do not give sufficient thought to how to implement the needed change.

Changes in hospitals and universities usually begin with some problem or challenge needing to be addressed. AI-based innovations may be proposed with buy-in from some level of administration after they have weighed matters, but too often the implementation of the idea is insufficiently addressed. Often inadequate attention is paid to preparing all concerned for the change, meaning all the stakeholders, including patients and their families. The generators of the proposed innovation are convinced of the need for change, in part because they have attended many meetings discussing the proposed change, but not enough attention is paid to communicating the need for the change to implementers of the change and to linking alterations to institutional mission. Too often administrators and experts forget all that they did to arrive at a decision and the individuals who will have to implement that decision have not been subject to the same indoctrination. The change process begins with "making sense" of the need for the change. Ideally this is done by connecting the new approach to longstanding values and a time-honored commitment to excellence, so the fresh tactic does not seem disassociated from what is familiar.

Preparing for the change is likely to mean new hires, obtaining other new resources, and training of those individuals who will be implementing the change. In environments full of providers and educators who are highly educated, it is particularly important that "not knowing some new technology" never gets depicted as a personal limitation because well-educated professionals do not want to feel as if their preparation is being impugned. Focus instead on the fact that the change will require all concerned to prepare for the needed change because the group is committed to quality. Leadership in this instance involves creating a culture of technologic proficiency, fostering an environment that embraces and encourages the use of technology, including AI [9]. It is also important that the proposed change be presented as an augmentation to existing practices, not a replacement for social connection, since AI is too often feared because it is artificial intelligence and not human intelligence.

The change process involves not only implementing the agreed-upon AI-based innovation but then monitoring that the new way of doing things remains consistent over time. Expect some relapses and make it easy for those implementing the change to let you know what goes wrong so you can address emerging difficulties in a timely fashion. Sometimes it is politically wise to refer to the innovation as a pilot study because those who are not enamored with the proposed changes are reminded that adoption of the innovation is dependent on it being an improvement over existing practice. Part of the initial plan should include expectations for hoped-for outcomes, so that data can be collected along the way, and the innovation is evaluated before becoming more widely adopted. Keep in mind that scaling up the innovation may require new organizational structures, controls and reward structures [10].

It is important to remember that an important part of the change process is celebrating success. What does this include above and beyond those involved getting together to rejoice in what they have accomplished? It means sharing successful outcomes with relevant administrators and stakeholders via personal communications, annual reports, websites, stories in the local community newspaper, and other media. It means describing what was accomplished at key professional meetings and in appropriate journals so other caregivers and educators can learn from your experiences. One of the biggest roles leaders play is touting the success of those who made possible the successful innovation. This cheerleading is important because success tends to beget additional achievement.

Outlook and Conclusions

Harkening back to President Biden's farewell address when he warned about the "profound possibilities and risks" that come with artificial intelligence, AI has the potential to improve human decision making by providing decision recommendations and problem-relevant information to assist healthcare professionals. But we need to better understand when the performance of a healthcare provider with AI assistance exceeds the performance of an unassisted provider or the AI help in isolation. Another concern is the timing of AI assistance and the amount of information to be presented to the decision maker for fear of cognitive overload and/or over-reliance on AI strategies [11]. It is those concerns and others not yet articulated that healthcare leaders must keep front and center.

What is clear is that IT/AI basics must be integrated into all leadership-development programs. In every career stage no matter what the specialty or setting, healthcare professionals must know enough to ask the IT/AI experts relevant questions: Why is this a situation in which AI should be leveraged? Do the proposed changes exceed current practices? Is the decision maker getting just the right amount of AI assistance or is the provider overwhelmed by the information received? Are there any unintended consequences resulting from the AI assistance? Providing care in a highly technological environment is challenging, particularly for novices who may be inclined to let technology draw all their attention rather than what is going on in the patient [12]. While AI assistance is most effective in data-driven decision-making and administrative tasks, it currently lacks the emotional intelligence of the human connection so healthcare leaders must know enough to choose wisely which innovations to espouse [13].

Useful Resources

American Academy of Nursing. Meeting's proceedings: addressing the challenges and policy implications of virtual nursing. 2024. https://aannet.org/page/virtual-nursing-2024.

American Academy of Nursing. AI transformation in policy, practice & education for nursing & health care: a foundational dialogue. 2024. https://aannet.org/events/eventdetails.aspx?id=1898565.

American Academy of Nursing. Meeting's proceedings: more than documentation burden creating burnout: what systems must do to achieve safe, efficient patient care using technology. 2023.

Perry AF, Federico F, Huebner J. Telemedicine: ensuring safe, equitable, person-centered virtual care. Boston: Institute for Healthcare Improvement; 2021. https://www.ihi.org/resources/white-papers/telemedicine-ensuring-safe-equitable-person-centered-virtual-care.

Review Questions

1. What are the three major views of leadership that surfaced in last century?
2. Name the five career stages discussed in this paper.

3. What are some of the IT/AI tasks that need to be addressed in the first career stage, Preparation?
4. What do the concepts—leadership and innovation—have in common?
5. What are some of the steps in the change process?

Answers to Review Questions

1. What are the three major views of leadership that surfaced in last century?
   (a) Leadership as personal—the ability to inspire and catalyze others
   (b) Leadership as achieving institutional mission—effectively meeting goals and wished-for outcomes
   (c) Leadership as getting ready for tomorrow—innovatively addressing challenges resulting from an evolving context
2. Name the five career stages discussed in this paper.
   (a) Preparation
   (b) Independent Contributions
   (c) Development of Home Setting
   (d) Development of Field/Health Care
   (e) Gadfly (Wise Person) Stage
3. What are some of the IT/AI tasks that need to be addressed in the first career stage, Preparation?
   (a) Information literacy
   (b) Computer competencies
   (c) Use of information management systems
   (d) Data analysis
   (e) Accessing and using evidence-based information
   (f) Using data for research and development
   (g) Using virtual assistants
   (h) Basics of cybersecurity
4. What do the concepts—leadership and innovation—have in common?
   (a) Innovation and leadership are concepts that have much in common because both are concerned with inspiring and catalyzing others to achieve institutional mission by designing new ways of achieving long-held values and goals.
5. What are some of the steps in the change process?
   (a) Establishing a need for the proposed change
   (b) Assembling the group who will lead the effort
   (c) Developing and communicating the plan
   (d) Encouraging new behaviors and risk taking
   (e) Communicating with stakeholders
   (f) Implementing and evaluating changes made
   (g) Hardwiring new systems
   (h) Celebrating successes

References

1. Liptak K, Forrest J, Sangal A, Hammond E. Key lines from President Joe Biden's farewell address. CNN; 2025. https://www.cnn.com/2025/01/15/politics/key-lines-from-president-joe-bidens-farewell-address/index.html.
2. McBride AB. The growth and development of nurse leaders. 2nd ed. New York: Springer; 2019.
3. Benner P. From novice to expert. Menlo Park. 1984;84:10–1097.
4. Dalton GW, Thompson PH, Price RL. The four stages of professional careers—a new look at performance by professionals. Organ Dyn. 1977;6:19–42.
5. Hübner U, Shaw T, Thye J, Egbert N, Marin HDF, Chang P, et al. An international recommendation framework of core competencies in health informatics for nurses. Technology Informatics Guiding Education Reform – TIGER. Methods Inf Med. 2018;57:e30–42.
6. Accreditation Council for Graduate Medical Education. Clinical informatics milestones. 2022. https://www.acgme.org/globalassets/pdfs/milestones/clinicalinformaticsmilestones.pdf.
7. American Psychological Association. Companion checklist: evaluation of an AI-enabled clinical or administrative tool. 2024. https://www.apaservices.org/practice/business/technology/tech-101/evaluating-artificial-intelligence-tool-checklist.pdf?utm_source=apa.org&utm_medium=referral&utm_content=/monitor/2025/01/trends-harnessing-power-of-artificial-intelligence.
8. Huang C, Zhang Z, Mao B, Yao X. An overview of artificial intelligence ethics. IEEE Trans Artif Intell. 2022;4:799–819.
9. Rony MKK, Parvin MR, Ferdousi S. Advancing nursing practice with artificial intelligence: enhancing preparedness for the future. Nurs Open. 2024;11:10.1002/nop2.2070.
10. Fihn SD, Saria S, Mendonça E, Hain E, Matheny M, Shah N, et al. Deploying AI in clinical settings. In: Artificial intelligence in health care: the hope, the hype, the promise, the peril. Washington, DC: National Academy of Medicine; 2020.
11. Steyvers M, Kumar A. Three challenges for AI-assisted decision-making. Perspect Psychol Sci. 2024;19:722–34.
12. Crilly G, Dowling M, Delaunois I, Flavin M, Biesty L. Critical care nurses' experiences of providing care for adults in a highly technological environment: a qualitative evidence synthesis. J Clin Nurs. 2019;28:4250–63.
13. Mohanasundari SK, Kalpana M, Madhusudhan U, Vasanthkumar K, Rani B, Singh R, et al. Can artificial intelligence replace the unique nursing role? Cureus. 2023;15:e51150.

Chapter 5
Implementation Science for AI Projects

Jan-David Liebe and Ursula H. Hübner

Learning Objectives

- To understand the role of implementation science in integrating AI into healthcare.
- To describe how logic models structure the planning and evaluation of AI implementations.
- To apply the Implementation Research Logic Model (IRLM) to AI implementation projects.
- To analyze barriers and facilitators and to identify suitable implementation strategies.
- To develop initial ideas for evaluating outcomes using appropriate metrics.
- To know complementary implementation frameworks.
- To understand basic ideas of human-centered implementation principles to the deployment of AI in healthcare settings.

Key Terms

- Implementation Science
- Logic Models
- Implementation Research Logic Model (IRLM)
- Barriers and Facilitators
- Implementation Outcomes

J.-D. Liebe (✉)
School of Business Management and Social Sciences, Osnabrück University of Applied Sciences, Osnabrück, Germany

UMIT - Private University of Health Sciences, Medical Informatics and Technology, Hall in Tirol, Austria
e-mail: j.liebe@hs-osnabrueck.de

U. H. Hübner
School of Business Management and Social Sciences, Osnabrück University of Applied Sciences, Osnabrück, Germany

U. H. Hübner et al. (eds.), *Bridging Artificial and Human Intelligence*, Health Informatics, https://doi.org/10.1007/978-3-032-11938-4_5

Summary
This chapter emphasizes the systematic approach required for AI implementations in healthcare settings. It introduces key implementation science frameworks, such as the Implementation Research Logic Model (IRLM), and explores how these models differentiate between determinants, implementation strategies, mechanisms of change, and measurable outcomes. The chapter explains the added value of logic models for the effective deployment of AI-driven applications, illustrating how these models help structure and operationalize implementation pathways. It provides examples of the different components and causal linkages within such frameworks and offers an outlook on how IRLM can enhance the scientific rigor, reproducibility, and evaluation of AI implementations in healthcare. Additionally, it presents complementary frameworks which analyze barriers, facilitators, and sustainability in AI adoption. Finally, the chapter introduces the idea of human-centered implementation science to facilitate sustainable AI uptake in clinical practice.

Implementation Science as a Framework for AI Integration

Although artificial intelligence in healthcare holds potential for advancements, its widespread implementation remains a challenge. Recent reviews of the current state of research reveal that only a few AI applications have progressed beyond experimental use in clinical practice [1]. The barriers to implementation are well documented and include both general factors that influence the adoption of health information technologies—such as integration into existing workflows, acceptance by professionals, and regulatory requirements—and challenges specific to AI, including the lack of interpretability of AI decisions, uncertainties regarding model reliability, and concerns about data protection and ethical responsibility [2].

Although these obstacles are well-documented, the main challenge is the development of structured methodologies that translate existing knowledge into effective implementation strategies. Thus, the challenge is not only to transfer AI into clinical practice but also to translate the existing knowledge about success factors and barriers into actionable strategies. Logic models provide a suitable framework for this process, as they help structure and operationalize implementation pathways in a systematic and evidence-based manner [3].

To systematically design and evaluate the implementation of AI in healthcare, this chapter adopts an implementation science perspective. Implementation science is a relatively recent field dedicated to facilitating the structured integration of evidence-based practices (EBPs) into routine healthcare with the aim of enhancing service quality and effectiveness [4, 5]. It acknowledges the persistent gap between research findings and their practical application, underlining that demonstrating effectiveness alone does not ensure adoption [5]. A key element within this field is the use of logic models, which provide a structured framework for planning, executing, and assessing implementation efforts [6].

Logic Models in Implementation Science

Traditional logic models offer a structured representation of program components by mapping resources, activities, and expected outcomes, which aids in planning and evaluation. For instance, in AI implementation, logic models can outline key inputs such as training programs and infrastructure adjustments, linking them to expected clinical and operational benefits. A classic logic model (often structured as *Inputs, Activities, Outputs, Outcomes*) helps stakeholders articulate how planned actions will lead to desired short- and long-term outcomes [7]. By mapping these connections, logic models simplify complex programs and clarify the assumed *theory of change*—i.e. the causal pathway by which an intervention is expected to bring about change [3, 8]. In implementation efforts, this approach facilitates decision makers to explicitly align their activities with outcomes, identify gaps or assumptions, and build an understanding of how an intervention should work. Logic models are used in program planning, implementation, and evaluation as they help to track progress and surface where and why a program succeeds or fails [3]. In contrast to traditional approaches, logical models can be read from the end to the beginning (upstream) instead of from the beginning to the end (downstream) thus focusing on the desired results tracing their path back step by step to the roots of the success. They essentially serve as a *"blueprint"* of an initiative, enhancing communication among stakeholders and guiding systematic evaluation from process and usage measures (outputs) to outcomes [7]. For example, if a dental clinic seeks to increase the patients' regular checkups in oral healthcare through a sophisticated personalized AI app (outcome), implementers should ensure that the app is used (output). This may entail measures to help patients use the system (activity 1) and motivate the use through education to become more familiar with their own health and their specific health risks (activity 2). These measures may then depend on the already existing or missing health literacy of the patients (input 1). In addition, to unfold its power, the algorithm of the app requires current data on the patient's eating habits, comorbidities and medication. Implementers must make sure that relevant interfaces to the patient's electronic health record are capable of routing through the necessary information (input 2) and that the patients are willing and able to regularly share eating habits and other lifestyle information (input 3). If these upstream steps are neglected the dental clinic may arrive at the conclusion that this new AI supported app is worthless even though it works perfectly well under ideal circumstances. This example only glimpses at the complexities of success and failure factors and points to the need to further refine the fabric of logic models.

Transition to the Implementation Research Logic Model (IRLM)

While traditional logic models set the stage, implementing evidence-based innovations in real-world settings often requires additional layers of detail [3]. Many frameworks in implementation science focus on specific aspects—for example, determinant frameworks (e.g. CFIR [9]) catalog context **barriers and facilitators**, while other models address implementation strategies or outcomes [3]. In practice, projects sometimes used multiple disparate models and failed to clearly justify how context, actions, and results fit together. The **Implementation Research Logic Model (IRLM)** was developed with the intention to bridge this gap by combining these elements into one integrated model [3]. Unlike a generic program logic model, the IRLM explicitly incorporates key implementation science constructs—*Determinants* (contextual factors), *Implementation Strategies*, *Mechanisms of Change*, and *Outcomes*—all in one framework. It prompts researchers and practitioners to specify the presumed relationships between these components, adding rigor and transparency to the logic of an implementation project. This approach offers added value: by making the causal pathways and assumptions explicit, the IRLM improves scientific rigor, reproducibility, and the ability to test how and why an implementation succeeds. In essence, IRLM extends the traditional logic model to not only say *"what we plan to do"* but also *"why and under what conditions it should work"*. It thereby provides a structured **roadmap** for implementation efforts [3].

Key Components of the Implementation Research Logic Model

The IRLM breaks down an implementation plan into interrelated components, each addressing a specific question about the project's logic:

- **Determinants:** Determinants are contextual factors that influence the success or failure of an implementation effort by acting as either barriers or facilitators. A key question in this regard is: Which contextual factors (e.g., organizational structures, provider readiness, patient engagement) impact the likelihood of successful implementation? Identifying these determinants (e.g. resource constraints, stakeholder commitment, or alignment with existing workflows) helps clarify where support is needed and where potential risks to adoption may arise [3]. In our example, time constraints of healthcare professionals to provide patient education on oral health and their motivation to share their data would act as barriers.
- **Implementation Strategies:** Implementation strategies are targeted actions designed to facilitate the implementation of an innovation by addressing identified barriers and leveraging facilitators [3]. In the IRLM framework, each strat-

egy should directly correspond to a specific determinant. Here, the central question is: What implementation tactics can be employed to mitigate barriers and strengthen facilitators? Strategies may include training programs, workflow integration, stakeholder engagement, policy adjustments, or financial incentives, each selected to address specific challenges. Powell et al. (2015) provide a refined compilation of 73 implementation strategies based on expert consensus [10] The IRLM emphasizes specifying who will implement these strategies, what actions will be taken, and why—ensuring a clear, evidence-based rationale for each approach [11]. In the example, time constraints for providing education could be mitigated by imparting education only to persons with low levels of health literacy and to those who would be willing to share their data with the app but face barriers that prevent them doing so. Additionally, further educational steps could be integrated into the app itself.

- **Mechanisms:** Mechanisms are the processes, mediators, or events that explain how an implementation strategy leads to change. They clarify the causal link between a strategy and its intended outcomes [3]. A key question in this context is: How will the chosen strategies generate the desired effects? Through what processes or behavioral changes will they influence outcomes? For example, if a strategy involves training clinicians on a new AI tool, a relevant mechanism might be increased clinician knowledge and confidence, which in turn promotes sustained tool usage. The IRLM framework emphasizes that mechanisms can manifest as shifts in determinant factors, such as an improved organizational climate, or as proximal changes (e.g. evolving user attitudes). Clearly defining these mechanisms helps assess whether an implementation strategy functions as intended and supports future refinements [3]. Referring to the example, it needs to be factored in that education alone may not work to change behavior. A thorough theoretical underpinning ensuring the use of the app is therefore worth considering. According to the Fogg Behavior Model, for example, motivation, ability and triggers play a major role in behavior change. The dental clinic may therefore prioritize those patients who shared data and used the app which may serve as a motivator, while education would act as an enabler.
- **Outcomes:** The Implementation Research Logic Model (IRLM) categorizes outcomes into implementation, service, and recipient (clinical) outcomes. Implementation outcomes assess the immediate effects of an intervention, such as adoption rates, fidelity, and acceptability [3]. Service outcomes measure its impact on healthcare delivery, including efficiency, quality of care, and safety. Recipient outcomes focus on direct patient or population health effects, such as improved diagnostics, treatment outcomes, or reduced hospitalizations. The main question is: Which quantitative and qualitative indicators can be used to assess the effectiveness of AI implementation, including factors such as adoption rates, user satisfaction, and long-term clinical benefits? For example, tracking the adoption and sustained use of an AI decision-support tool (implementation), its effect on workflow efficiency (service), and improvements in diagnostic accuracy (recipient) ensures a comprehensive evaluation of both process and impact. In the case of the AI app example, implementation outcome is represented by the

usage rate of the app, the service outcome is reflected by the number of checkups and the clinical outcome finally can be measured by a change (decrease) in the rate of dental problems.

Tables 5.1, 5.2, 5.3, 5.4, 5.5, and 5.6 present the elements of the IRLM along different levels in detail, i.e. patient and workforce level, organizational level and macro level.

The IRLM components are interconnected, with explicit links between them. It clarifies which determinants each strategy addresses, which mechanisms the strategy activates, and how these mechanisms lead to specific outcomes. This structured mapping makes the model both a planning tool and a testable hypothesis (e.g., "Implementing Strategy X to address Barrier Y will trigger Mechanism Z, leading to Outcome O") [3]. Figure 5.1 illustrates a logic model in terms of the IRLM for implementing AI in healthcare.

Table 5.1 Determinants

Level	Determinant	Description
Patient and workforce-level	Trust in AI-driven care	Patients are more likely to accept AI-driven healthcare solutions if they perceive them as trustworthy, explainable, and aligned with human decision-making [12]. Low AI literacy and fears about data security can act as barriers [13].
	AI literacy and clinician trust	Healthcare professionals may lack training in AI and may also struggle to interpret AI-generated recommendations, leading to skepticism [14]. Fear of liability and clinical responsibility concerns can also hinder adoption [15].
Organizational-level	Workflow compatibility and interoperability	AI must seamlessly integrate into EHRs to reduce clinician workload, while mitigating ethical risks related to bias, privacy, and security in clinical summarization [16]. Poor interoperability with existing IT infrastructure is a key barrier for AI implementation [17].
	Leadership and institutional commitment	Strong leadership support, clear AI governance policies, and investment in AI-friendly infrastructure increase adoption. Resistance from administrators or unclear policies can slow implementation [18].
Macro-level	Regulatory uncertainty and liability risks	Clear and well-defined AI regulations, liability frameworks, and compliance standards provide legal certainty, fostering investment, adoption, and responsible AI implementation in healthcare [19]
	Economic incentives and reimbursement models	Adequate reimbursement models and financial incentives from insurance companies, governments, and hospital administrators can encourage AI adoption by demonstrating cost-effectiveness and long-term value [20].

Table 5.2 Implementation strategies

Level	Implementation strategy	Description
Patient and workforce-level	AI literacy and patient engagement programs	Providing patient-friendly AI explanations, ensuring transparency in AI decision-making, and facilitating informed consent builds trust and encourages patient engagement with AI-driven healthcare solution [21].
	Clinician AI education and decision-support training	Structured AI training programs and decision-support simulations help clinicians understand AI outputs, reducing skepticism and increasing responsible use [14].
Organizational-level	Seamless AI integration into clinical workflows	Embedding AI systems into EHRs, hospital IT infrastructure, and decision-support pathways to ensure efficient adoption, reduce cognitive burden on clinicians, and address ethical considerations such as transparency, fairness, and data security [16, 17].
	Strong leadership and AI governance policies	Institutions leadership should establish clear AI governance structures, create multidisciplinary AI task forces, and provide institutional support for AI projects to ensure responsible implementation, foster collaboration, and address ethical and regulatory considerations [18].
Macro-level	Regulatory standardization and liability frameworks	Governments and regulatory bodies must develop clear liability frameworks and standardized compliance guidelines for AI in healthcare to reduce uncertainty [19].
	Financial incentives and reimbursement mechanisms	Policymakers and payers should develop AI reimbursement models and value-based incentives to encourage adoption and ensure sustainability [20].

Table 5.3 Implementation mechanisms

Level	Implementation mechanism	Description
Patient and workforce-level	Increased transparency and trust-building	AI literacy and engagement programs increase patient understanding, fostering trust and acceptance of AI-generated healthcare insights [12, 13].
	Cognitive alignment and decision augmentation	AI training enables clinicians to align AI insights with medical reasoning, reducing resistance and promoting responsible decision-making [14].
Organizational-level	Reduced cognitive load and workflow efficiency	AI systems that are seamlessly embedded into EHRs and clinical workflows reduce manual workload and decision fatigue for clinicians [16, 17].
	AI accountability and institutional trust	Strong institutional leadership and clear AI governance policies ensure that clinicians understand responsibility for AI decisions, reducing liability concerns [18].

(continued)

Table 5.3 (continued)

Level	Implementation mechanism	Description
Macro-level	Legal certainty and risk mitigation	Regulatory standardization and liability frameworks reduce legal risks, encouraging hospitals and clinicians to safely adopt AI [19].
	Economic feasibility and sustainability	Reimbursement models and value-based incentives make AI adoption financially sustainable, promoting long-term integration [20].

Table 5.4 Implementation outcomes

Level	Implementation outcome	Description
Patient and workforce-level	Patient acceptance of AI tools	The degree to which patients feel comfortable using AI-driven tools for healthcare decision-making and self-management [22].
	Clinician adoption and sustained use of AI	The extent to which clinicians integrate AI into their workflow and continue using it over time [23].
Organizational-level	Successful AI system integration	The effectiveness of embedding AI into the healthcare institutions IT infrastructure and workflows, ensuring minimal disruptions [24].
	AI governance and compliance adherence	The ability of healthcare institutions to establish AI oversight structures, regulatory compliance, and accountability measures [25].
Macro-level	Regulatory approval and legal acceptance	The extent to which AI systems receive formal regulatory approval and align with legal and ethical guidelines [18].
	Economic viability and financial sustainability	The long-term financial feasibility of AI adoption, including return on investment, cost savings, and reimbursement feasibility [18].

Table 5.5 Service outcomes

Level	Service outcome	Description
Patient and workforce-level	Improved patient engagement and self-management	AI-powered remote monitoring and decision-support tools help patients actively participate in their care [26].
	Reduction in clinician workload and burnout	AI-driven automation of administrative tasks and clinical decision support reduces cognitive burden on healthcare providers [16, 27].
Organizational-level	Increased hospital workflow efficiency	AI enhances resource allocation, triage, and scheduling, leading to improved operational efficiency [28, 29].
	Higher accuracy in clinical decision-making	AI-assisted diagnostics and treatment planning can contribute to more precise and data-driven medical decisions [30].

(continued)

Table 5.5 (continued)

Level	Service outcome	Description
Macro-level	Improved population health monitoring and early disease detection	AI-based predictive analytics help detect outbreaks, track disease trends, and optimize public health responses [31].
	Enhanced healthcare system responsiveness	AI for improving system resilience in healthcare (e.g. emergency response coordination, telemedicine infrastructure, and supply chain logistics) [32].

Table 5.6 Recipient outcomes

Level	Recipient outcome	Description
Patient and workforce-level	Better health outcomes and quality of life	AI-driven personalized medicine, early diagnostics, and predictive analytics lead to improved patient health and well-being [33].
	Increased clinician decision confidence and decreased interrater variability	AI assisted decision making in advanced cancer therapy can result in greater confidence in the decision and in decreased variability among the clinicians [34]
Organizational-level	Reduction in medical errors and adverse events	Machine Learning prediction model outperformed statistical scores in predicting major adverse events in the cardiac intensive unit, i.e. death, resuscitated cardiac arrest, cardiogenic shock, and helped risk stratification of patients [35].
	Better patient-provider communication and shared decision-making	LLM could generate better material for patient education and shared decision making compared to the one from existing sources [36]
Macro-level	Reduction in healthcare disparities and equitable access	As a scoping review recommended training data for AI models should amongst other improve diversity, quality and quantity of data, evaluated disparities in model performance, use equity-focused checklists, guidelines and similar tools [37].
	Sustainable health system cost reduction	A cost simulation based on real values for colorectal cancer incidence rates and mortality with and without AI screening resulted in cost reductions due to reduced rates with AI screening [38].

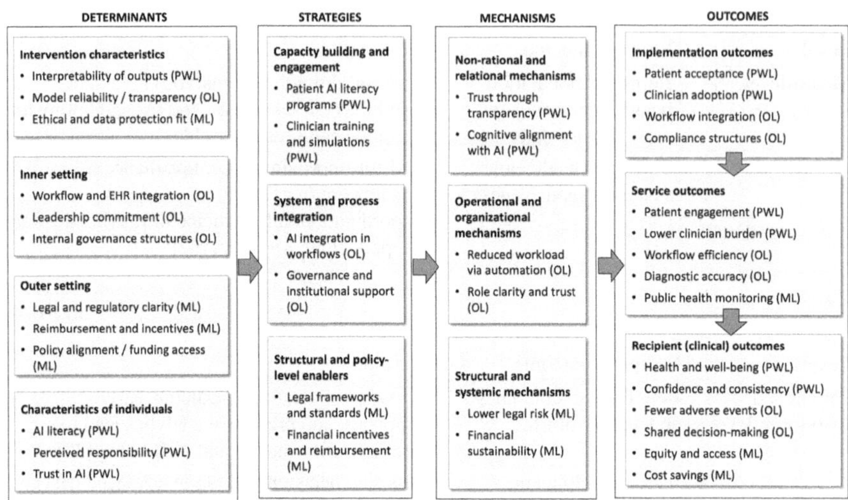

Fig. 5.1 Example of an IRLM for AI in healthcare. Legend: PWL patient and workforce level, OL organizational level, ML macro level

Practical Example: IRLM Applied to Healthcare AI Implementation

The Implementation Research Logic Model (IRLM) provides a structured approach to integrating AI in healthcare, ensuring that implementation is systematic and effective. A case study by Baxter et al. illustrates this process with a machine-learning model designed to predict hospital readmissions from critical variables such as age, diagnoses, laboratory values, medication types, current length of stay, past emergency department visits, and past hospitalizations. The prediction model outperformed the risk score that was widely used before [39]. The team first identified key determinants affecting adoption, such as workflow variability, clinician unawareness of the tool, and hesitancy due to reliance on the older risk score. Additionally, users questioned the tool's relevance and highlighted the need for proper training. To address these challenges, the team developed implementation strategies, including early stakeholder engagement, targeted training, and workflow integration to improve clinician acceptance and ensure seamless adoption. The underlying mechanism focused on closing knowledge gaps and improving workflow compatibility in order to improve clinicians' confidence and encourage sustained use. The expected outcome was higher adoption of the AI model in routine care, ultimately leading to reduced hospital readmissions and improved patient outcomes [39].

This example highlights the value of the IRLM in guiding AI implementation. By explicitly linking strategies to determinants, mechanisms, and outcomes, the model paves the way for a logical and evidence-based approach to adoption. In this way, the IRLM serves both as a planning tool and an evaluation framework, supporting AI interventions become successfully implemented and deliver measurable improvements in healthcare [3].

Complementary Role of Other Implementation Frameworks

While logic models like the IRLM provide a structured approach to implementation planning, other frameworks offer complementary insights by analyzing the contextual factors that influence success. The NASSS framework examines why digital health innovations fail to scale, focusing on technological complexity, stakeholder dynamics, and systemic barriers [40]. The CFIR framework identifies key determinants of implementation, such as organizational readiness and external influences, making it particularly useful for understanding barriers and facilitators [9]. The RE-AIM framework evaluates implementation across multiple dimensions, including reach, adoption, and long-term sustainability, offering a broader perspective on an intervention's impact [41]. Rather than excluding each other mutually, these frameworks complement logic models by bridging contextual analysis with structured implementation planning. While NASSS, CFIR, and RE-AIM help identify potential challenges and success factors, logic models like the IRLM translate these insights into actionable implementation strategies. Using them in combination offers both a comprehensive understanding of implementation barriers and a systematic approach to overcoming them.

Implementing AI with a People-First Approach: Human-Centered Implementation Science

Successful AI implementation requires a human-centered approach, ensuring that integration aligns with clinical workflows, addresses user needs, and incorporates iterative adaptation based on user feedback. Human-centered implementation science extends the ethos of user-centricity into the process of integration and uptake [42] This means that when rolling out an AI system in a healthcare setting, implementers prioritize user needs, workflow integration, training, and organizational culture just as much as technical installation [43]. Key principles for a human centered AI approach are:

- **Meeting Users Where They Are:** Rather than expecting clinicians or staff to radically change their routines to accommodate the AI application, the implementation adapts the AI software to fit into existing routines and systems. This involves workflow integration (e.g., embedding AI alerts into the electronic health record interface that providers already use, or timing AI outputs to align with clinical decision points dispersed over the day). Failure to integrate into the workflow is a known barrier; studies have found that AI tools not woven into clinicians' normal processes quickly fall by the wayside [44]. A human-centered rollout might pilot the AI system in one department to gather feedback on workflow fit, adjust the tool's triggers or interface based on that feedback, and only then scale up. Throughout this process, maintaining clinician autonomy is crucial—the AI application should support, not override the professional's judgment [44].

- **Training and Support:** No matter how well-designed an AI system is, users need to understand what it does, how it works, and why it is useful. Implementation plans should include robust education and training. This can range from formal training sessions to on-demand quick reference guides and responsive IT support. The goal is to build users' confidence and competence in using the AI tool. For example, introducing an AI sepsis early warning system might involve hands-on training for nurses and physicians, emphasizing not just the technical steps (how to access the alert dashboard) but also why the system can improve patient outcomes [45]. Such training can build trust and reduce anxiety by clarifying that the AI is there to assist. In one real-world deployment, implementers noted that comprehensive training and communication about the AI's purpose and workflow were essential in preparing frontline staff and ensuring smooth adoption [45]. Ongoing support is also part of human-centered implementation—users should have channels to ask questions or report issues (for instance, a helpdesk or regular check-ins by the implementation team).
- **Champion Engagement and Leadership Buy-In:** Human-centered implementation pays attention to the social dynamics of change. Identifying and empowering clinical "champions" (e.g. respected end-users who advocate for the AI tool) can accelerate adoption. Champions help communicate benefits to peers and can mentor colleagues in early use. Studies have highlighted that having clinician leaders involved from the onset and visibly endorsing the AI application can drive buy-in [44]. Similarly, organizational leadership support (hospital executives, department heads) is important to allocate resources and signal that the change is valued. When both frontline and leadership stakeholders are on board, resistance diminishes. Champions and opinion leaders essentially serve as human touchpoints that contextualize the AI system for others, share success stories, and address skepticism with peer-to-peer communication [18].
- **Iterative Adaptation and Feedback Loops:** A key aspect of human-centered implementation is treating deployment as an iterative process rather than as a one-time event. This requires mechanisms to systematically collect user feedback and performance data, allowing for continuous refinement of the system and its integration into workflows. Effective strategies include debrief meetings after pilot phases, monitoring usage patterns and outcomes, and establishing accessible feedback channels, such as surveys for clinicians [45]. Continuous evaluation helps address technical and usability challenges while fostering engagement and trust among users. For example, in one AI deployment, regular meetings with nurses and physicians identified workflow misalignments, leading to modifications in alert escalation pathways to better fit clinical roles. Such adaptability promotes a continuous responsiveness of the implementation to user needs, ultimately aiming at the effectiveness and long-term sustainability within the clinical environment.

Outlook and Conclusions

While logic models, implementation science and human-centered design are not new they play a role of paramount importance when the mere technology seems to overwhelm its implementers and users. In such cases these approaches guide the perspective towards the context in which the implementation takes place and help remind all stakeholders that the humans are the ones who bring meaning to the application of the technology.

Today many AI applications appear so stunning that the attention often solely rests on what the application can achieve and how much better it performs a single task than humans. Therefore, a context and user driven mindset seems even more needed to lead the implementation process to a clinically meaningful success. The past decades have witnessed great failures when seeking to put grand technology plans into practice, e.g. national eHealth strategies. In these cases, the agency of the technology was much less intrusive and interfering than today's AI applications which come with a larger portion of risks, also risks of failure. To make these AI applications successful the environment they are embedded in must be factored in when implementing them. The measures taken may be similar to those for other technologies, but their ultimate impact may even be more crucial due to the potential effect of the AI system—both in terms of harms and benefits. There is a strong need to evaluate the overall performance of AI systems that can be guided by logical models and their pathways toward the impact of the system. Thus, context and human-centered designs also taking ethical considerations into account may build the bridge between artificial and human intelligence during implementation and evaluation.

Useful Resources

The Implementation Research Logic Model (IRLM): The video provides an overview of the IRLM and its application in planning and evaluating implementation projects: https://www.youtube.com/watch?v=BBI9BYvKC2I

Implementation Research Logic Model (IRLM) Overview: Comprehensive guide to the IRLM, including tools and templates for developing your own logic models: https://hivimpsci.northwestern.edu/implementation-research-logic-model/

Review Questions

1. What is the Implementation Research Logic Model (IRLM) , and how does it differ from traditional logic models?
2. How can logic models support the structured implementation of AI in healthcare settings?
3. What are common barriers to AI adoption in clinical practice, and how can they be addressed using implementation strategies?
4. How do complementary frameworks (NASSS, CFIR, RE-AIM) enhance AI implementation planning?

5. What key principles can be considered in a human-centered approach to AI implementation?

Answers to Review Questions

1. The Implementation Research Logic Model (IRLM) extends traditional logic models by explicitly incorporating key implementation science constructs: determinants, implementation strategies, mechanisms of change, and outcomes. Unlike generic logic models, IRLM links these components systematically, improving the transparency, reproducibility, and evaluation of implementation efforts.
2. Logic models help structure AI implementation by offering a framework that maps out the relationships between key factors such as resources, actions, and outcomes. They enable stakeholders to identify potential gaps, align strategies with intended results, and ensure a systematic approach to planning and evaluation.
3. Common barriers to AI adoption include lack of workflow integration, clinician skepticism, regulatory uncertainty, and ethical concerns. These challenges can be addressed through targeted implementation strategies such as AI literacy training, seamless system integration, stakeholder engagement, and clear governance policies.
4. Complementary frameworks provide additional insights into AI implementation. The NASSS framework identifies systemic barriers to scaling digital innovations, CFIR helps analyze organizational readiness and external influences, and RE-AIM evaluates the long-term sustainability and impact of an intervention. These frameworks complement logic models by bridging contextual analysis with structured implementation planning.
5. A human-centered approach to AI implementation prioritizes user needs and workflow integration. Key principles include adapting AI to existing clinical routines, providing comprehensive training and support, engaging clinical champions and leadership, and maintaining iterative feedback loops to continuously refine AI deployment based on user experience.

References

1. Yin J, Ngiam KY, Teo HH. Role of artificial intelligence applications in real-life clinical practice: systematic review. J Med Internet Res. 2021;23:e25759. https://doi.org/10.2196/25759.
2. Ahmed MI, Spooner B, Isherwood J, Lane M, Orrock E, Dennison A. A systematic review of the barriers to the implementation of artificial intelligence in healthcare. Cureus. 2023;15:e46454. https://doi.org/10.7759/CUREUS.46454.
3. Smith JD, Li DH, Rafferty MR. The implementation research logic model: a method for planning, executing, reporting, and synthesizing implementation projects. Implement Sci. 2020;15:1–12. https://doi.org/10.1186/S13012-020-01041-8/TABLES/1.
4. Eccles MP, Mittman BS. Welcome to implementation science. Implement Sci. 2006;1:1–3. https://doi.org/10.1186/1748-5908-1-1/METRICS.

5. Bauer MS, Damschroder L, Hagedorn H, Smith J, Kilbourne AM. An introduction to implementation science for the non-specialist. BMC Psychol. 2015;3:1–12. https://doi.org/10.1186/S40359-015-0089-9/TABLES/5.
6. Czosnek L, Zopf EM, Cormie P, Rosenbaum S, Richards J, Rankin NM. Developing an implementation research logic model: using a multiple case study design to establish a worked exemplar. Implement Sci Commun. 2022;3:1–12. https://doi.org/10.1186/S43058-022-00337-8/FIGURES/2.
7. Savaya R, Waysman M. The logic model. Adm Soc Work. 2005;29:85–103. https://doi.org/10.1300/J147V29N02_06.
8. Mclaughlin JA, Jordan GB. Using logic models. In: Handbook of practical program evaluation. 4th ed. Wiley; 2015. p. 62–87. https://doi.org/10.1002/9781119171386.CH3.
9. Damschroder LJ, Reardon CM, Opra Widerquist MA, Lowery J. Conceptualizing outcomes for use with the consolidated framework for implementation research (CFIR): the CFIR outcomes addendum. Implement Sci. 2022;17:1–10. https://doi.org/10.1186/S13012-021-01181-5/TABLES/2.
10. Powell BJ, et al. A refined compilation of implementation strategies: results from the expert recommendations for implementing change (ERIC) project. Implement Sci. 2015;10:1–14. https://doi.org/10.1186/S13012-015-0209-1/TABLES/3.
11. Smith JD, Li DH, Rafferty MR. The implementation research logic model: a method for planning, executing, reporting, and synthesizing implementation projects. Implement Sci. 2020;15:84. https://doi.org/10.1186/S13012-020-01041-8.
12. Esmaeilzadeh P, Mirzaei T, Dharanikota S. Patients' perceptions toward human–artificial intelligence interaction in health care: experimental study. J Med Internet Res. 2021;23:e25856. https://doi.org/10.2196/25856.
13. Shevtsova D, et al. Trust in and acceptance of artificial intelligence applications in medicine: mixed methods study. JMIR Hum Factors. 2024;11:e47031. https://doi.org/10.2196/47031.
14. Asan O, Bayrak AE, Choudhury A. Artificial intelligence and human trust in healthcare: focus on clinicians. J Med Internet Res. 2020;22:e15154. https://doi.org/10.2196/15154.
15. Nair M, Svedberg P, Larsson I, Nygren JM. A comprehensive overview of barriers and strategies for AI implementation in healthcare: mixed-method design. PLoS One. 2024;19:e0305949. https://doi.org/10.1371/JOURNAL.PONE.0305949.
16. Lee C, Vogt KA, Kumar S. Prospects for AI clinical summarization to reduce the burden of patient chart review. Front Digit Health. 2024;6:1475092. https://doi.org/10.3389/FDGTH.2024.1475092.
17. Rehburg F, Graefe A, Hübner M, Thun S. How interoperability can enable artificial intelligence in clinical applications. Stud Health Technol Inform. 2024;316:596–600. https://doi.org/10.3233/SHTI240485.
18. Davenport TH, Glaser JP. Factors governing the adoption of artificial intelligence in healthcare providers. Discov Health Sys. 2022;1:4. https://doi.org/10.1007/S44250-022-00004-8.
19. Mennella C, Maniscalco U, De Pietro G, Esposito M. Ethical and regulatory challenges of AI technologies in healthcare: a narrative review. Heliyon. 2024;10:e26297. https://doi.org/10.1016/J.HELIYON.2024.E26297.
20. Venkatesh KP, Raza MM, Diao JA, Kvedar JC. Leveraging reimbursement strategies to guide value-based adoption and utilization of medical AI. NPJ Digit Med. 2022;5:112. https://doi.org/10.1038/S41746-022-00662-1.
21. Rosenbacke R, Melhus Å, McKee M, Stuckler D. How explainable artificial intelligence can increase or decrease clinicians' trust in AI applications in health care: systematic review. JMIR AI. 2024;3:e53207. https://doi.org/10.2196/53207.
22. Kelly S, Kaye SA, Oviedo-Trespalacios O. What factors contribute to the acceptance of artificial intelligence? A systematic review. Telematics Inform. 2023;77:101925. https://doi.org/10.1016/J.TELE.2022.101925.

23. Lambert SI, et al. An integrative review on the acceptance of artificial intelligence among healthcare professionals in hospitals. NPJ Digit Med. 2023;6:111. https://doi.org/10.1038/S41746-023-00852-5.
24. Rahimi AK, et al. Implementing AI in hospitals to achieve a learning health system: systematic review of current enablers and barriers. J Med Internet Res. 2024;26:e49655. https://doi.org/10.2196/49655.
25. Economou-Zavlanos NJ, et al. Translating ethical and quality principles for the effective, safe and fair development, deployment and use of artificial intelligence technologies in healthcare. J Am Med Inform Assoc. 2024;31:705–13. https://doi.org/10.1093/JAMIA/OCAD221.
26. Botha NN, et al. Artificial intelligent tools: evidence-mapping on the perceived positive effects on patient-care and confidentiality. BMC Digit Health. 2024;2:1–24. https://doi.org/10.1186/S44247-024-00091-Y.
27. Loftus TJ, et al. Artificial intelligence and surgical decision-making. JAMA Surg. 2020;155:148–58. https://doi.org/10.1001/JAMASURG.2019.4917.
28. Knight DRT, et al. Artificial intelligence for patient scheduling in the real-world health care setting: a metanarrative review. Health Policy Technol. 2023;12:100824. https://doi.org/10.1016/J.HLPT.2023.100824.
29. Boonstra A, Laven M. Influence of artificial intelligence on the work design of emergency department clinicians a systematic literature review. BMC Health Serv Res. 2022;22:1–10. https://doi.org/10.1186/S12913-022-08070-7/FIGURES/2.
30. Lam TYT, Cheung MFK, Munro YL, Lim KM, Shung D, Sung JJY. Randomized controlled trials of artificial intelligence in clinical practice: systematic review. J Med Internet Res. 2022;24:e37188. https://doi.org/10.2196/37188.
31. El Morr C, Ozdemir D, Asdaah Y, Saab A, El-Lahib Y, Sokhn ES. AI-based epidemic and pandemic early warning systems: a systematic scoping review. Health Informatics J. 2024;30:14604582241275844. https://doi.org/10.1177/14604582241275844.
32. Arji G, Ahmadi H, Avazpoor P, Hemmat M. Identifying resilience strategies for disruption management in the healthcare supply chain during COVID-19 by digital innovations: a systematic literature review. Inform Med Unlocked. 2023;38:101199. https://doi.org/10.1016/J.IMU.2023.101199.
33. Ali O, Abdelbaki W, Shrestha A, Elbasi E, Alryalat MAA, Dwivedi YK. A systematic literature review of artificial intelligence in the healthcare sector: benefits, challenges, methodologies, and functionalities. J Innov Knowl. 2023;8:100333. https://doi.org/10.1016/J.JIK.2023.100333.
34. Niraula D, et al. Intricacies of human–AI interaction in dynamic decision-making for precision oncology. Nat Commun. 2025;16:1–19. https://doi.org/10.1038/s41467-024-55259-x.
35. Weizman O, et al. Machine learning score to predict in-hospital outcomes in patients hospitalized in cardiac intensive care unit. Eur Heart J Digital Health. 2025;6:218–27. https://doi.org/10.1093/EHJDH/ZTAE098.
36. Shah YB, Ghosh A, Hochberg A, Mark JR, Lallas CD, Shah MS. Artificial intelligence improves urologic oncology patient education and counseling. Can J Urol. 2024;31(5):12013–8. Available: https://www.canjurol.com/html/subscriber/Spdf/V31I05/CJU_V31I5_10_DrShah.pdf.
37. Thomas Berdahl C, Lawrence Baker S, Mann OO, Girosi F. Strategies to improve the impact of artificial intelligence on health equity: scoping review. JMIR AI. 2023;2:e42936. https://doi.org/10.2196/42936.
38. Areia M, et al. Cost-effectiveness of artificial intelligence for screening colonoscopy: a modelling study. Lancet Digit Health. 2022;4:e436–44. https://doi.org/10.1016/S2589-7500(22)00042-5.
39. Baxter SL, Bass JS, Sitapati AM. Barriers to implementing an artificial intelligence model for unplanned readmissions. ACI Open. 2020;04:e108–13. https://doi.org/10.1055/S-0040-1716748.

40. Greenhalgh T, et al. Beyond adoption: a new framework for theorizing and evaluating non-adoption, abandonment, and challenges to the scale-up, spread, and sustainability of health and care technologies. J Med Internet Res. 2017;19:e367. https://doi.org/10.2196/JMIR.8775.
41. Glasgow RE, Vogt TM, Boles SM. Evaluating the public health impact of health promotion interventions: the RE-AIM framework. Am J Public Health. 2011;89:1322–7. https://doi.org/10.2105/AJPH.89.9.1322.
42. Waddell A, et al. Leveraging implementation science in human-centred design for digital health. Conference on Human Factors in Computing Systems – Proceedings. 2024;24:17. https://doi.org/10.1145/3613904.3642161/SUPPL_FILE/3613904.3642161-TALK-VIDEO.VTT.
43. Chen E, Neta G, Roberts MC. Complementary approaches to problem solving in healthcare and public health: implementation science and human-centered design. Transl Behav Med. 2021;11:1115–21. https://doi.org/10.1093/TBM/IBAA079.
44. Hassan M, Kushniruk A, Borycki E. Barriers to and facilitators of artificial intelligence adoption in health care: scoping review. JMIR Hum Factors. 2024;11:e48633. https://doi.org/10.2196/48633.
45. Sendak MP, et al. Real-world integration of a sepsis deep learning technology into routine clinical care: implementation study. JMIR Med Inform. 2020;8:e15182. https://doi.org/10.2196/15182.

Part III
Case Studies

Chapter 6
Artificial Intelligence in Dermatology

Usman Iqbal, Long-Chen (Tommy) Li, and Yu-Chuan (Jack) Li

Learning Objectives

- To understand dermatology as an example of visual medicine
- To understand how AI transformed dermatology
- To describe how an AI-based tool in dermatology can look like and what it can achieve
- To explain future developments and advances of the application of AI in dermatology to improve patient care
- To understand the special and general ethical concerns in dermatology

Key Terms

- Image based diagnostics
- Skin cancer classification
- Automated disease classification
- Predictive analytics
- Tele-dermatology
- Future developments
- Ethical concerns

Summary

The integration of artificial intelligence (AI) into dermatology represents a transformative shift in modern medicine. The past decade has witnessed significant advancements in AI algorithms designed for dermatological applications, particularly in

U. Iqbal
Bond University, Gold Coast, Australia

L.-C. (Tommy) Li
Johns Hopkins University, Baltimore, USA

Y.-C. (Jack) Li (✉)
Taipei Medical University, Taipei, Taiwan
e-mail: jack@tmu.edu.tw

U. H. Hübner et al. (eds.), *Bridging Artificial and Human Intelligence*, Health Informatics, https://doi.org/10.1007/978-3-032-11938-4_6

image-based diagnosis and automated disease classification. This chapter presents the MoleMe case study. MoleMe, launched in 2019 by a team of dermatologists and AI researchers in Taiwan, is an AI-powered skin monitoring application designed to analyze moles and lesions for early signs of malignancy that has been used by more than 200,000 users. To fully realize its promise, future efforts must prioritize algorithmic accuracy, dataset inclusivity, and seamless integration into clinical workflows.

Introduction

The integration of artificial intelligence (AI) into dermatology represents a transformative shift in modern medicine. Dermatology, a field heavily reliant on visual pattern recognition for diagnosing conditions like skin cancer, eczema, and psoriasis, is uniquely suited to benefit from AI's image analysis capabilities. AI algorithms, particularly those leveraging deep learning and convolutional neural networks (CNNs), have demonstrated remarkable accuracy in classifying skin lesions, predicting treatment outcomes, and enhancing tele-dermatology platforms [1, 2]. This integration promises to improve diagnostic accuracy, streamline workflows, and enhance patient access to care, especially in underserved areas [3]. This chapter explores the current applications, challenges, and future potential of AI in dermatology, supported by clinical evidence and ethical considerations.

AI's rapid evolution in dermatology is driven by its ability to process and analyse vast amounts of image data, making it an ideal technology for a specialty that is visual in its diagnostic process [4]. The chapter delves into the evolution of AI applications in dermatology over the past decade, covering key advancements and use cases, such as the development of MoleMe, an AI-powered dermatology mobile app developed for consumers to determine the risk of pigmented moles, which demonstrates how AI can support both patients and clinicians [5, 6].

Literature Review: AI in Dermatology Over the Past Decade

The past decade has witnessed significant advancements in AI algorithms designed for dermatological applications, particularly in image-based diagnosis and automated disease classification (Fig. 6.1).

Image-Based Diagnosis

AI-powered systems, particularly deep learning models, have demonstrated diagnostic capabilities comparable to those of dermatologists in detecting conditions like melanoma and other skin cancers. For example, deep learning outperformed

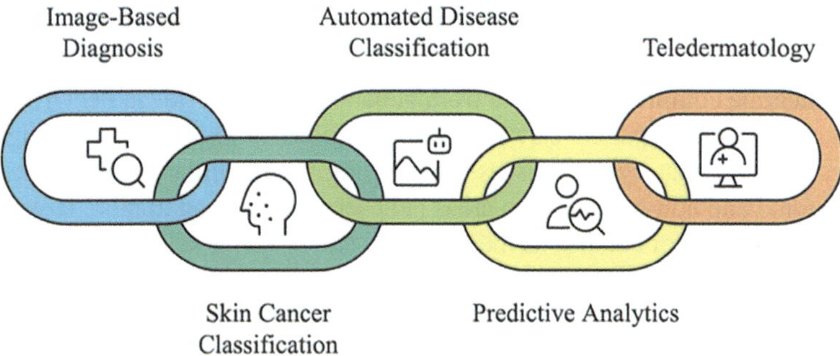

Fig. 6.1 Transforming dermatology with artificial intelligence

136 of 157 dermatologists in a head-to-head task classifying dermoscopic melanoma images, underscoring AI's potential in clinical diagnostics [7]. CNNs trained on dermoscopic images have shown promise in improving early detection rates [1], and studies suggest AI-assisted diagnosis can enhance clinician performance while reducing unnecessary biopsies [8].

Dermatologist-Level Classification of Skin Cancer with Deep Neural Networks

Skin cancer, the most common human malignancy, is primarily diagnosed visually, and automated classification of skin lesions is a challenging task due to their fine-grained variability. In a study, Esteva et al. (2017) demonstrated that a CNN, trained on a dataset of 129,450 clinical images across 2032 diseases, performed on par with 21 board-certified dermatologists in classifying two critical skin cancer types. This demonstrated AI's ability to classify skin cancer at a level comparable to dermatologists, offering the potential for mobile devices to extend dermatological diagnostics beyond clinical settings [1].

Automated Disease Classification

AI has also shown promise in diagnosing a range of other skin diseases, including eczema, psoriasis, and fungal infections [9]. These models improve diagnostic accuracy, especially in busy clinical settings. A study by Tschandl et al. (2019) highlighted that machine learning algorithms outperformed human experts in classifying pigmented skin lesions, emphasizing the potential of AI to augment diagnostic accuracy in clinical practice, particularly in conditions with high variability [10]. However, AI models still face challenges when exposed to out-of-distribution images, underscoring the need for further development in this area.

Predictive Analytics and Personalized Treatment

Machine learning models can predict treatment outcomes based on patient history, genetic markers, and environmental factors, enhancing personalized care [11]. AI-powered platforms, such as those recommending personalized skincare regimens, integrate comprehensive data from genetic tests, lifestyle, and environmental exposures to optimise patient care [12]. Recent studies have explored gene signature profiles in inflammatory skin diseases, unveiling unique inflammatory patterns in both lesional and non-lesional skin areas [11], which may lead to more targeted and early interventions for conditions like psoriasis and systemic sclerosis. Furthermore, the Baumann Skin Typing System (BSTS) and AI-driven routines are revolutionising personalized skincare, offering tailored solutions for diverse concerns like acne prevention and anti-aging. These AI-powered systems, based on large datasets, enable dermatologists to craft customised skincare regimens for patients, improving patient outcomes by ensuring treatments address specific skin types [12].

Tele-dermatology and AI-Enabled Remote Consultations

AI-driven tele-dermatology platforms are transforming dermatological care delivery, particularly in underserved regions. These platforms allow clinicians to remotely assess skin lesions, facilitating timely and accurate diagnoses without the need for patients to travel long distances. Machine learning and computer vision technologies power these systems, helping primary care physicians and nurse practitioners improve their diagnostic decision-making [13]. Studies show that AI-assisted diagnosis increases agreement between primary care physicians and reference dermatologists, improving diagnostic accuracy by up to 12% and reducing unnecessary referrals and biopsies [13, 14].

Use Case: MoleMe—Taiwan's AI Dermatology Innovation

Background and Development

MoleMe, launched in 2019 by a team of dermatologists and AI researchers in Taiwan, is an AI-powered skin monitoring application designed to analyze moles and lesions for early signs of malignancy that has been used by more than 200,000 users. Leveraging deep learning and image recognition, MoleMe aims to provide consumers with a simple tool to determine the risk of pigmented skin moles as a mobile app on smart phones (as shown in Fig. 6.2), facilitating the early detection of skin issues for quicker interventions and improved outcomes [5, 6].

ASKiN ENG
Responses from operator
Please Select AI Evaluation Item (Free)
Immediately evaluate the dangerous sign of your skin health by uploading a photo and answering some questions!
Evaluate Acne
Evaluate Mole
Evaluate Nail (Beta version)
Online Doctor Consultation
Reserve
AI Health Evaluation
Evaluate Now
Record
My Voucher
Customer Service Center
Service Menu
ASKiN ENG
Responses from operator
I'm MoleMe, mastering in making people know the risk of their moles. Nice to meet you!
I've evaluated thousands of moles. By answering some questions and uploading a picture of mole, you can get the result.
Furthermore, you can watch the video related to moles filmed by dermatologists!
Take or upload a photo of the acne you want to analyze. Please refer to the example photo and the reminders below.
Use the back camera to take
Online Doctor Consultation
Reserve
AI Health Evaluation
Evaluate Now
Record
My Voucher
Customer Service Center
Service Menu
MoleMe
Online Doctor Consultation
in one image, please frame one first. Thank you!)
Frame your mole
Got the photo! Next, answer 5 simple questions to make the analysis more accurate!
How long has the mole been existing as you know?
About 1 month
About a year
More than 1 year
Reserve
AI Health Evaluation
Evaluate Now
Record
My Voucher
Customer Service Center
Service Menu
a month? For example: getting bigger, discoloring, deforming, bleeding, being painful or itchy.
I'm not sure
Almost finished! Does the size of the mole larger than 0.6cm?
No
What is your age range?
Under 21 years old
21-40 years old
41-65 yea
Lower
Lower Risk
Based on the result, please refer to the following videos.
Instructions
Avoid Mole Lesions

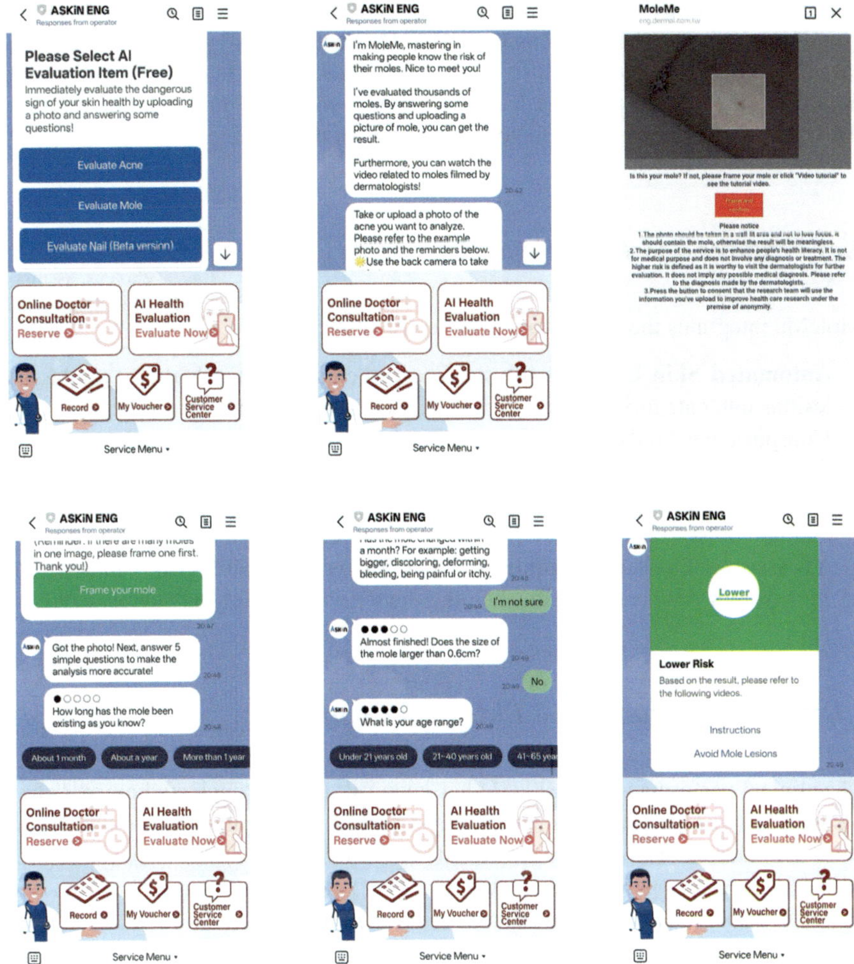

Fig. 6.2 Snapshots from the MoleMe (ASKiN) app showing the evaluation steps of a mole case

The creation of MoleMe was a response to the increasing incidence of skin cancer and the need for more accessible and reliable tools for skin health monitoring. As skin cancer remains one of the most prevalent cancers globally, early detection is crucial for improving survival rates. MoleMe combines dermatological expertise with AI to deliver a convenient solution that allows individuals to take a quick photo of their moles using their own smart phones. The AI core was trained using more than 30,000 of mole images taken by consumers while the risk was determined by board-certified dermatologists as ground truth. Each original image was spawned into 20 derived images with different lighting, background hues, sizes and angles before feeding into the machine-learning engine to make the training more robust to the skin tones and also to the photo-taking skills of the users.

Key Features and Functionality

MoleMe integrates the following AI-driven functionalities:

- **Automated Skin Lesion Analysis**: The app employs deep learning to classify lesions into categories of benign, suspicious, or malignant.
- **Comparative Analysis**: Users can upload images over time to track changes in moles and other skin abnormalities.
- **Integration with Telemedicine**: MoleMe facilitates remote consultations with dermatologists, enabling timely expert reviews of concerning images.
- **AI-Assisted Decision Support for Clinicians**: Dermatologists can also use MoleMe for AI-based insights, helping them prioritise high-risk cases.

Clinical Performance and Physician Comparison

The clinical performance of MoleMe has been validated through studies, including a significant comparison with human physicians. A study published in the British Journal of Dermatology [5] demonstrated that MoleMe's AI model achieved an area under the receiver operating characteristic (ROC) curve (AUC) of 0.94, which outperforms most general practitioners (GPs) in classifying the risk of cutaneous pigmented lesions.

Furthermore, the AI model showed a sensitivity of 0.96 and a specificity of 0.87. Sensitivity indicates the AI's ability to correctly identify true positive cases (e.g., higher risk lesions), while specificity refers to its ability to identify true negative cases (e.g., lower risk lesions). These high values underscore the reliability of MoleMe as a screening tool for higher risk pigmented moles.

In addition, a user satisfaction study revealed that over 90% of users were satisfied with the app's usability and its positive impact on daily life [6]. This high satisfaction rate highlights MoleMe's widespread acceptance across demographics. Its accessibility and ease of use contribute to its growing popularity, and its potential to help prioritising access to dermatological care is substantial.

Challenges and Future Developments

Despite its success, MoleMe faces several important challenges:

- **Regulatory Hurdles**: AI-powered medical tools like MoleMe must undergo rigorous validation, clinical testing, and approval processes before widespread deployment. Regulatory frameworks tend to favour high-resource environments, creating barriers for global implementation, particularly in low- and middle-income countries [15]. The lack of tailored regulations for AI adds further uncertainty.
- **Bias and Generalizability**: If AI models are trained on datasets that lack diversity in skin tones, ages, and sociodemographic backgrounds, diagnostic accuracy may be compromised. Most AI training data comes from western countries and most skin images used in dermatology textbooks were Type I (white) skin [16]. This lack of diversity can perpetuate health inequities and reduce the reliability of the tool for underserved populations [17]. Enhancing inclusivity in dataset curation and spawning the original images with different lighting, background, skin tone, view angles, etc. can also reduce the risk of biases. It is crucial to conduct sufficient external validations during the model evaluation processes to avoid over-fitting.
- **Integration with Healthcare Systems**: For MoleMe to reach its full potential, it should be integrated into the pre-visit process of primary care practices. Such integration would enhance clinical decision-making, and care coordination [18, 19]. However, challenges related to interoperability, data privacy, and clinician trust must be navigated carefully [20].

Addressing these challenges will bring MoleMe as well as similar AI tools closer to fulfilling their potential as an accessible, accurate, and equitable digital dermatology solution.

Comparative Analysis of AI Dermatology Tools

Table 6.1 compares MoleMe [5] with other notable AI-driven dermatology applications i.e., DermEngine [21] and SkinVision [20].

Table 6.1 Benchmarking MoleMe with other AI-driven dermatology applications

Feature	MoleMe	DermEngine	SkinVision
AI diagnosis	Yes	Yes	Yes
Mobile app	Yes	Yes	Yes
Teledermatology	Yes	Yes	No
Regulatory approval	Pending	Approved	Approved
Data training diversity	Moderate	High	Moderate

Outlook: The Future of AI in Dermatology

The evolution of AI in dermatology can be categorized into four distinct stages:

1. **Predictive (Perception) AI**
   Current AI applications in dermatology largely function as predictive tools that analyse medical images to detect patterns and classify skin conditions. These models rely on deep learning algorithms trained on large datasets to achieve diagnostic accuracies comparable to expert dermatologists [22]. AI systems can classify lesions such as melanoma and other skin cancers, enabling early detection and improving patient outcomes.
   In cosmetic dermatology, predictive AI tools are also emerging to offer objective assessments of aesthetic concerns. These models can evaluate skin texture, pigmentation, and symmetry, assisting dermatologists in creating personalised treatment plans [23]. AI's data-driven insights complement the subjective evaluations traditionally used in aesthetic practice, enhancing both clinical decision-making and patient satisfaction.
   Looking ahead, developments in predictive AI may focus on refining real-time image analysis, integrating seamlessly with clinical workflows and electronic health records. However, patient trust remains a critical barrier. While patients are open to AI-supported diagnoses, many require the technology to surpass dermatologist-level accuracy or, in the worst case scenario, when the healthcare cost is so unbearable, before accepting AI-only assessments [22]. Future models must therefore prioritise transparency, explainability, and continuous validation to support broader clinical adoption.
2. **Generative AI in Dermatology**
   Generative AI, particularly models such as generative adversarial networks (GANs) and generative pre-trained transformer (GPT) are changing dermatological practice and research. These models can synthesise realistic skin lesion images, thereby enriching training datasets and mitigating the scarcity of annotated images especially for underrepresented skin tones [24, 25]. Beyond image generation, generative AI enables simulation of disease progression, supporting dermatologist training and patient education by visualising how nevi may evolve into melanomas [25]. Such innovations align with traditional diagnostic frameworks, like the ABCDE rule, to enhance early skin cancer detection and personalised care.
   Moreover, generative AI models can inform treatment planning by simulating therapeutic responses over time, offering a dynamic approach to personalised dermatological interventions [26]. This capability complements recent work demonstrating the promise of large language models (LLMs) like ChatGPT in providing accurate second opinions on dermatological diagnosis and treatments, though limitations persist in medication coding and specificity [27]. Despite these advances, equity in AI training data remains critical; without inclusive datasets, generative tools risk reinforcing existing health disparities in dermatology [26].

3. **Agentic AI in Dermatology**

   Agentic AI represents a shift from passive decision-support tools to systems capable of actively guiding dermatological care. Emerging models aim to autonomously navigate clinical workflows, synthesising multimodal patient data to recommend treatments or diagnostic actions with minimal human intervention [28, 29]. These agentic systems promise enhanced efficiency and access, particularly in underserved regions, where dermatological expertise is limited. However, their deployment must be critically evaluated to ensure alignment with clinician values and professional autonomy elements central to dermatologists' identity and sensemaking around AI adoption [29].

   For instance, while AI-powered chatbots such as ChatGPT have shown capacity to simplify dermatological information and triage basic queries, concerns remain over diagnostic reliability, misinformation, and the risk of over-standardisation [30]. As AI tools become more autonomous, rigorous clinical validation and ethical safeguards are essential to mitigate potential harms. The profession must navigate tensions between efficiency and care quality, and between broader access and the preservation of patient–clinician relationships.

   Ultimately, agentic AI could redefine dermatological practices, but not replace clinical expertise—provided it is implemented through transparent, equitable, and culturally sensitive frameworks [28, 31].
4. **Physical AI: The Role of Humanoid Robots in Dermatology**

   As AI continues to evolve, its physical embodiment in the form of humanoid robots presents exciting possibilities for dermatology. Moving beyond virtual tools and software, future applications may include AI-integrated robots capable of conducting dermatological assessments through a combination of advanced image recognition and tactile sensing [32]. These robots could replicate human-like interactions and even interventions while maintaining high levels of diagnostic precision.

   In cosmetic dermatology, automated robotic devices are already being explored to assist hair transplant [33] and energy-based treatments, such as laser resurfacing and mole removal, with promising prospects for enhanced procedural consistency and patient outcomes [32]. The integration of artificial skin technologies and anthropomorphic features further refines these robots' ability to simulate human touch and appearance, enhancing patient comfort and engagement [34].

   However, challenges remain regarding the psychological acceptance of humanoid robots, particularly in relation to the "uncanny valley effect", as well as ensuring ethical, safe interaction in clinical settings [34]. As the technology matures, physical AI may become a valuable adjunct in both cosmetic and clinical dermatology, augmenting physician capabilities and expanding patient access to precise, technology-assisted care.

Ethical and Systematic Considerations

Despite AI's promising advancements in dermatology, challenges remain in ensuring its effective and ethical integration. One key concern is the need for more diverse datasets to ensure AI systems can accurately diagnose skin conditions across different skin tones. Han et al. (2018) highlighted that AI models trained on more inclusive datasets especially those representing individuals with various skin tones will be more effective in providing accurate diagnoses for a global population [35]. Furthermore, the integration of AI into clinical workflows must balance the technology's capabilities with the indispensable role of human practitioners in patient care [36, 37].

Algorithmic bias remains a concern, as AI systems have demonstrated suboptimal performance on out-of-distribution images [10]. To address this, the development of AI models that can generalise across diverse datasets is essential for ensuring their reliability and effectiveness in real-world clinical settings. Without inclusivity in training datasets, AI tools risk perpetuating existing disparities in dermatological care. Therefore, prioritising diverse and representative datasets is essential to mitigate bias and improve diagnostic accuracy across all demographics.

While AI has considerable potential in dermatology, its integration must be done carefully. Topol (2019) asserts that AI should augment, not replace, human judgement in healthcare, while Norgeot et al. (2019) advocate for "smarter healthcare systems" that allow AI to continuously learn from electronic health records, personalising care delivery [36, 37]. Moreover, the use of AI in tele-dermatology raises ethical challenges, such as the potential exacerbation of health disparities due to a lack of standardised regulations or informed consent protocols [3].

Ethical concerns in AI's dermatological applications also include issues like misdiagnosis, data security, privacy violations, and the risk of replacing human jobs [3]. To ensure the responsible deployment of AI in dermatology, key ethical principles such as fairness, inclusivity, transparency, accountability, and privacy must be prioritised. These principles should guide the development and implementation of AI tools, addressing concerns around equity and accuracy in diagnosis and care delivery [3].

Outlook and Conclusions

In our use case, MoleMe offers a practical, AI-powered solution for early skin cancer detection. By combining clinical and image data, it exemplifies the shift towards patient-centred, AI-driven dermatology. With clinical performance surpassing that of many general practitioners and high user satisfaction, MoleMe holds strong potential as a vital tool in global skin health.

AI is driving a transformative shift in dermatological diagnostics, from predictive analytics to generative and embodied intelligence, dermatology stands on the brink of transformative change. While challenges persist particularly around regulatory frameworks and dataset diversity ongoing innovation continues to refine AI's clinical utility. To fully realize its promise, future efforts must prioritize algorithmic accuracy, dataset inclusivity, and seamless integration into clinical workflows.

Useful Resources

TMU spin-off DermAI's robot recognizes 90% of abnormal moles. https://oge.tmu.edu.tw/tmu-spin-off-dermais-robot-recognizes-90-of-abnormal-moles/

Artificial Intelligence in Dermatology: A Comprehensive Review of Approved Applications, Clinical Implementation, and Future Directions. https://pubmed.ncbi.nlm.nih.gov/40387622/

Review Questions

Here are some examples:

1. What are the five transformative forces in advancing AI in dermatology?
2. What are features of AI-based tools such as MoleMe?
3. What are challenges for AI-based tools such as MoleMe?
4. What are future perspectives of AI in dermatology?
5. What are ethical concerns of using AI in dermatology?

Answers to Review Questions

1. AI in dermatology was shaped by image-based diagnosis, skin cancer classification with deep neural networks, automated disease classification, tele-dermatology including AI-enables remote consultations and predictive analytics in combination with personal treatment.
2. The example of MoleMe shows that AI tools can comprise skin lesion analytics to classify them into severity classes, comparative analyses over time, provide tele-medicine consultation and AI assisted decision support for clinicians.
3. Despite its success MoleMe was confronted with challenges such as regulatory hurdles, bias and generalizability due to the dataset used and integration into the workflows of the healthcare system.
4. The future of AI in dermatology will be influenced by advances in predictive analytics, generative AI and its application in dermatology, actively guiding clinicians in dermatological care and physical AI where robots analyze skin images and conduct tactile sensing to offer diagnostic and treatment recommendations.
5. Ethical concerns arise from reduced generalizability due to datasets that are not divers enough and therefore lead to systems that are not performing very well in out-of-distribution images. This might result in perpetuating existing disparities. Further concerns arise from the need to establish a balanced interaction between clinicians and the AI system that supports the clinical workflows and does not aim at replacing clinicians. On top of this, there are general ethical issues such as data security, potential privacy violations and accountability.

References

1. Esteva A, et al. Dermatologist-level classification of skin cancer with deep neural networks. Nature. 2017;542:115–8.
2. Liu Y, et al. A deep learning system for differential diagnosis of skin diseases. Nat Med. 2020;26:900–8.

3. Gordon ER, et al. Ethical considerations for artificial intelligence in dermatology: a scoping review. Br J Dermatol. 2024;190:789–97.
4. Hogarty DT, et al. Artificial intelligence in dermatology—where we are and the way to the future: a review. Am J Clin Dermatol. 2020;21:41–7.
5. Chin Y, et al. A patient-oriented, general-practitioner-level, deep-learning-based cutaneous pigmented lesion risk classifier on a smartphone. Br J Dermatol. 2020;182:1498–500.
6. Chin YPH, et al. User satisfaction with a smartphone-compatible, artificial intelligence-based cutaneous pigmented lesion evaluator. Comput Methods Prog Biomed. 2020;195:105649.
7. Brinker TJ, et al. Deep learning outperformed 136 of 157 dermatologists in a head-to-head dermoscopic melanoma image classification task. Eur J Cancer. 2019;113:47–54.
8. Haenssle HA, et al. Man against machine: diagnostic performance of a deep learning convolutional neural network for dermoscopic melanoma recognition in comparison to 58 dermatologists. Ann Oncol. 2018;29:1836–42.
9. Zhang Y, et al. Current views on neuropeptides in atopic dermatitis. Exp Dermatol. 2021;30:1588–97.
10. Tschandl P, et al. Comparison of the accuracy of human readers versus machine-learning algorithms for pigmented skin lesion classification: an open, web-based, international, diagnostic study. Lancet Oncol. 2019;20:938–47.
11. Martínez BA, et al. Machine learning reveals distinct gene signature profiles in lesional and nonlesional regions of inflammatory skin diseases. Sci Adv. 2022;8:eabn4776.
12. Baumann L. AI-guided personalized skin care and custom routines. J Cosmet Sci. 2024;75:e82510.
13. Jain A, et al. Development and assessment of an artificial intelligence–based tool for skin condition diagnosis by primary care physicians and nurse practitioners in teledermatology practices. JAMA Netw Open. 2021;4:e217249.
14. Giavina-Bianchi M, Santos AP, Cordioli E. Teledermatology reduces dermatology referrals and improves access to specialists. EClinicalMedicine. 2020;29:100641.
15. Price W, Nicholson I. Medical AI and contextual bias. Harv JL Tech. 2019;33:65.
16. Celi LA, et al. Sources of bias in artificial intelligence that perpetuate healthcare disparities—a global review. PLOS Digital Health. 2022;1:e0000022.
17. Franklin G, et al. The sociodemographic biases in machine learning algorithms: a biomedical informatics perspective. Life (Basel). 2024;14:652.
18. Aloysius C, et al. Teledermatology in primary care in Singapore: experiences of family doctors and specialists. Acta Derm Venereol. 2021;101:221.
19. Zakaria A, et al. Cost minimization analysis of a teledermatology triage system in a managed care setting. JAMA Dermatol. 2021;157:52–8.
20. Smak Gregoor AM, et al. An artificial intelligence based app for skin cancer detection evaluated in a population based setting. npj Digit Med. 2023;6:90.
21. Young AT, et al. The role of technology in melanoma screening and diagnosis. Pigm Cell Melanoma Res. 2021;34:288–300.
22. Wu A, Ngo M, Thomas C. Assessment of patient perceptions of artificial intelligence use in dermatology: a cross-sectional survey. Skin Res Technol. 2024;30:e13656.
23. Kania B, Montecinos K, Goldberg DJ. Artificial intelligence in cosmetic dermatology. J Cosmet Dermatol. 2024;23:3305–11.
24. Pillai J, Li B. Generative artificial intelligence in dermatology: recommendations for future studies evaluating the clinical knowledge of models. Skin Res Technol. 2024;30:e13854.
25. Jütte L, et al. Generative AI for enhanced skin cancer diagnosis, dermatologist training, and patient education. In: Photonics in dermatology and plastic surgery 2025. San Francisco: SPIE; 2025.
26. Adamson AS, Smith A. Machine learning and health care disparities in dermatology. JAMA Dermatol. 2018;154:1247–8.
27. Iqbal U, et al. Can large language models provide secondary reliable opinion on treatment options for dermatological diseases? J Am Med Inform Assoc. 2024;31:1341–7.

28. Du Crest D, et al. Skin and digital–the 2024 narrative. Mayo Clin Proc Digit Health. 2024;2:322–30.
29. May J, et al. 51070 artificial intelligence in dermatology: a sensemaking analysis. J Am Acad Dermatol. 2024;91:AB127.
30. Chen R, et al. The chatbots are coming: risks and benefits of consumer-facing artificial intelligence in clinical dermatology. J Am Acad Dermatol. 2023;89:872–4.
31. Wongvibulsin S, Lee I. Artificial intelligence and dermatology. JAMA Dermatol. 2025;161:344.
32. Elder A, et al. The role of artificial intelligence in cosmetic dermatology—current, upcoming, and future trends. J Cosmet Dermatol. 2021;20:48–52.
33. Rose PT, Nusbaum B. Robotic hair restoration. Dermatol Clin. 2014;32:97–107.
34. Minh Trieu N, Truong Thinh N. A comprehensive review: interaction of appearance and behavior, artificial skin, and humanoid robot. J Robot. 2023;2023:5589845.
35. Han SS, et al. Deep neural networks show an equivalent and often superior performance to dermatologists in onychomycosis diagnosis: automatic construction of onychomycosis datasets by region-based convolutional deep neural network. PLoS One. 2018;13:e0191493.
36. Topol EJ. High-performance medicine: the convergence of human and artificial intelligence. Nat Med. 2019;25:44–56.
37. Norgeot B, Glicksberg BS, Butte AJ. A call for deep-learning healthcare. Nat Med. 2019;25:14–5.

Chapter 7
Bridging Artificial Intelligence and Care—Smart Assistive Technologies for Long-Term Care

Katrin Lehner and Vera Gallistl-Kassing

Learning Objectives

- To understand which AI technologies are developed for and implemented in the long-term care sector
- To gain an understanding about the specific challenges of implementing AI in long-term care, particularly with regard to the views of care staff and older adults
- To identify methods for creating meaningful connections between care and AI, particularly through participatory design and responsible innovation practices
- To understand a conceptional framework that that considers care and AI as relational and in connection, instead of viewing them as separate spheres

Key Terms

- Older Adults,
- Ageing,
- AI-Ageism,
- AI-enriched Care Relations

Summary

Artificial intelligence (AI) is promoted as a solution for challenges in long-term care, but its implementation raises ethical concerns and practical difficulties. This chapter critically examines the co-constitution of aging and AI by analysing how AI technologies are contextualized in long-term care. Based on interviews with residents, care staff, and AI-developers, we explore three AI-systems *in context*: a fall-detection sensor, the social robot Pepper, and the robotic seal Paro. Our findings highlight three pathways towards AI-enriched care: (1) Involving older adults in AI development and implementation, (2) recognizing both human and technological

K. Lehner (✉) · V. Gallistl-Kassing
Center for Gerontology and Health Research, Karl-Landsteiner University of Health Sciences, Krems, Austria
e-mail: katrin.lehner@kl.ac.at; vera.gallistl@kl.ac.at

U. H. Hübner et al. (eds.), *Bridging Artificial and Human Intelligence*, Health Informatics, https://doi.org/10.1007/978-3-032-11938-4_7

vulnerabilities, and (3) fostering meaningful connections between older adults, care staff and AI. We argue that participatory approaches are crucial for bridging the gap between AI and care, ensuring more inclusive and ethical practices in AI-enriched long-term care.

Introduction

The adoption of artificial intelligence (AI) in long-term care has accelerated in response to growing demands for care efficiency and optimization in times of demographic change. Today, AI in long-term care is increasingly used in hopes of supporting health and care professionals in a variety of ways, and enabling older adults to live and age autonomously and independently [1, 23, 24]. In the last years, the market for AI in long-term care has significantly grown, with market research predicting savings up to eight billion Euro over the next decade in AI-based dementia diagnoses alone [22].

Ever since its first development in the 1990s, where the first automated monitoring systems for older adults in need of care have been developed, AI for elder care has vastly diversified. Today, AI in long-term care comprises decision support systems for medical diagnosis [2], automated analysis of patients' data for early disease detection and preventive medicine [2, 23], robotics to provide care support as conversational agents [24], or monitoring and surveillance systems for older adults living and ageing in place [15].

While the public discourse around AI in care is often focussed on its promising potentials, research has identified several challenges in the practical implementation of AI in long-term care. Scholars highlighted ethical concerns, including the automatization and depersonalization of care, as well as surveillance and discrimination against minorities [23] as challenges of AI in long-term care. Also, questions about the human dimensions of care, such as empathy, intuition and the consideration of nuanced patient needs, remain central to the debate [30]. Research also pointed out that ageism and age-discrimination influence the way AI is developed for care settings—particularly when older adults, their needs and voices are insufficiently represented in the AI development and implementation process [26, 27]. This "AI ageism" [26] refers to bias and exclusions in AI that disadvantage older adults through algorithms and datasets, stereotypes and prejudices in AI development and through a lack of representation of aging in AI discussions (among others) [27]. Studies have, for instance, documented that AI-systems for facial recognition are more prone to errors with faces of older adults [16], and highlighted that when AI-systems are implemented in long-term care, older adults are often not given sufficient information to actively engage with these complex technological systems—partly because of ageist stereotypes that portray older adults as uninterested or incompetent in relation to new technologies [12].

As a consequence, despite rapid advancements in AI development for the long-term care sector, many technologies face significant obstacles in practical implementation. Lukkien et al. [14] note that AI in long-term care and its related guidelines and practices of responsible innovation requires careful *contextualization*, meaning that AI-technologies must be adapted to the specific circumstances in which they are used in. This includes ethical frameworks and sensitivity to users' needs, to ensure AI is consistent with the complexity of long-term care, including older adults, their families and multiple health and care professionals. However, existing applications and guidelines often remain too abstract to enable genuine contextualization. Similarly, it has been noted more research is needed to explore how AI systems for older adults can be effectively and meaningfully integrated into existing care arrangements. This would provide a deeper understanding of their potential beyond techno-optimistic promises of efficiency and productivity gains [6]. At the centre of these promises lies a so called "techno-solutionism" [40], which assumes that social and structural challenges in care can be fixed through technological innovation alone. This lack of engagement between AI development and the long-term care sector is also problematized by Peine and Neven [21], who argue that research on care technology and ageing often follows an interventionist logic, that positions technologies as neutral "problem-solvers", designed to address predefined needs or assumed "problems" of ageing, while at the same time making the active engagement of older users with these technologies invisible. Following this argument, Hartmann et al. [38] point out the tendency of machine learning to standardise and normalise human behaviour, and thereby disregarding individual variability and reinforcing established norms of emotions and interactions. However, by framing AI as a solution a one-sided focus on technological efficiency is reinforced and its practical implementation in complex, dynamic and relational systems and networks of care are overlooked.

In this chapter, we want to challenge such simplified separations between AI and long-term care and instead follow calls by multiple scholars [6, 21] to consider, study and theorize the co-constitution of ageing and artificial intelligence, by asking how AI-systems are practically contextualized and appropriated in long-term care settings. Such a perspective challenges the widely used binary thinking that assumes technology and care as two separate and unrelated spheres, and instead asks how technologies and care practices are intertwined, come together, influence and shape each other. In the following, we share research findings from a project that explored the use and implementation of AI in long term care to ask how good care can be shaped in collaboration with artificial intelligence. Focussing our reflections on 'bridging' AI and long-term care, the chapter answers the following questions:

- How are AI technologies practically implemented and contextualized in the long-term care sector?
- Which challenges arise in this process, particularly with regards to differing logics of AI development and long-term care ("*separating AI and care*")?
- What is needed to successfully connect AI and long-term care ("*bridging AI and care*")?

Bridging AI and Long-Term Care—A Reflection Based on Three Examples

This chapter draws on results and data from the ALGOCARE project, which followed three AI technologies from its development towards its implementation in nursing homes: An AI-supported fall-detection sensor, the social robot "Pepper" and the robot seal "Paro". During this process, the project team conducted qualitative interviews with AI developers, care staff and older adults in need of care to understand the needs and challenges of diverse groups in the implementation process of AI in long-term care settings.

Data was collected from July to October 2022 and from November 2023 to January 2024. The studied facilities housed approximately 100–150 residents with varying levels of care needs. A total of 37 semi-structured interviews were conducted (Table 7.1).

Additionally, participant observations, focussing on daily routines within the care facilities and interactions involving the technologies, amounting to approximately 24 h were performed. Interview transcripts and observation notes were analysed using MAXQDA 2022 by a team of four researchers. The analysis was conducted through open coding, followed by collaborative sessions using situational analysis [5]. The analysis identified routines, practices, and power structures relevant to the practical implementation of AI technology in care settings, highlighting both factors that contribute to the separation and to opportunities of bridging long-term care and AI-technologies.

In the following chapters, we lay out the basic functions of the three studied AI-technologies and discuss potentials and challenges of each technology. After that, we share findings from the ALGOCARE project to discuss a) where AI and the practices of long-term care are made different and distinct from one another ("*separating*") and b) how AI can be blended into existing practices of care and enrich care practices ("*bridging*").

Table 7.1 Formative evaluation of three AI technologies in nursing homes: interviews

Perspective	Number of interviews
Care residents	10
Care staff	14
Care management	2
AI developers	11
Total number of interviews	**37**
Participant observations (in hours)	24

AI-Based Fall Detection Sensors

Fall detection and prevention, particularly through behaviour monitoring, is one key area of AI development for long-term care settings. Fall detection systems generally are implemented to monitor physical activities and movements of older adults, continuously analysing data to distinguish between daily routines and potential falls. While the increased risk of falls among older adults is often used as a key argument for the development and implementation of AI fall detection sensors [29], research shows that cost efficiency in care is a driving factor as well [8]. However, this economic efficiency is often accompanied with standardisation, resulting in less individualised care practices and the objectification of patients [39]. Fall detection and prevention systems typically monitor older adults' behaviour and alert care staff in case of a detected fall [28]. Additionally, some fall detection systems can use analysis of movement patterns to give insights into the health of residents and to inform preventative measures [10]. In the case of the AI-system studied in the ALGOCARE project, the fall detection system used 3D sensors to gather depth data about older adults' movement in their rooms. Based on machine learning algorithms, these sensors processed collected data to identify objects, individuals, and movements, and alert care staff in case of a fall. The system was installed in care home residents' rooms, operated continuously and provided round-the-clock monitoring.

Existing research on AI-based fall detection systems have identified several challenges in the development and implementation in long-term care. Literature highlights the lack of reliability and accuracy of fall detection systems. Some daily activities, such as sitting down on a chair, tying shoelaces and fitness exercises may be falsely identified as falls, leading to alarms and unnecessary disruption of the daily lives of residents and care routines [28]. Others documented challenges of obtaining authentic data in real-world scenarios, that is needed to train AI fall detection, as another key barrier [31], as data collection in long-term care settings is a challenging, cost-intensive and ethical issue. Also, privacy concerns, especially for sensors using visual data, are regularly highlighted in literature [31].

One major challenge in the implementation of this AI technology that became apparent in the ALGOCARE project was the unavailability of training data on older adults' falls. In the interviews, AI developers shared that their developed model would require large, diverse datasets to be trained and function effectively. However, real-world data of older populations, in particular of older adults falling, was seen to be hard to collect, as access to a large and diverse group of participants (e.g. older adults living in long-term care facilities) was seen as restricted. As a result, developers turned to alternative sources of data to train their AI model—highlighting the potentials of synthetic data, where data on falls was recorded not in real-time, but by AI developers putting on motion capture suits. These practices of synthetic data creation, however, also established a clear separation between AI development and long-term care, as AI developers would not routinely engage with the people and places their AI models were being developed for (see [7] for a deeper discussion on this issue). As a consequence, the voices and needs of older adults, were relatively absent in AI development process.

In our interviews with older adults living with the developed sensors, it became clear that residents engaged with the sensors in their room with curiosity and interest:

> *"At the beginning, you keep looking at it because it's new and you think 'Is it ever going to start?"*

Others shared that they would change and adapt their everyday practices to avoid false alarms or tried to engage with the sensors to find out what the system does. These results highlight the potential of bridging AI and care by recognising older adults not just as passive "vessels of data" but as active contributors to AI development and implementation. By taking older adult's existing interest in AI-technologies into account, their agency in the context of AI cam be addressed and supported [19].

The Humanoid Robot "Pepper"

Pepper is a 1.2-m-tall social robot with a friendly face, human-like body, moveable arms and fingers and wheels for mobility. It uses microphones, several sensors and 3D cameras for navigation, speech, hearing, object and face detection in order to tailor its contents to the respective user. Pepper has an integrated tablet on its chest, which is intended to help with communication and the display of customisable content, such as games and photos. While its hardware is produced by a major American company since 2014, smaller companies worldwide are responsible for selling and programming Pepper, focussed on individual applications and tailored functionalities depending on customers and fields of application [22].

For the long-term care sector, Obst et al. [20] pointed out that robotics is a complex and challenging field. Despite significant funding for care robot development, few robots are implemented in practice. Data protection and liability remain challenging, as ethical concerns about data collection, storage, and accountability for robot errors are unclear [20]. For Pepper specifically, Mishra et al. [18] tested functions of the robot and found issues with face recognition, navigation, and conversation accuracy. This miscommunication is also emphasized in studies on Pepper's interactions with older adults. Stommel et al. [25] observed miscommunication in all 36 interviews with older adults, particularly "trouble hearing" when the participant and robot spoke about each other, leading to repetition and frustration.

One central challenge of using Pepper in long-term care that became evident in the ALGOCARE project was that existing robots were hardly able to engage with caring practices in a person-centred way. One example for this lies in the entertainment that was provided by Pepper, which was often based on assumptions about older adults' needs, competences and preferences, rather than actual input by older adults. For example, the developer emphasises that the robot is able to present content according to a person's estimated age:

> *"And he [the robot] can then adjust his level accordingly based on the age and based on the overall facial expressions and gestures."*

While this function is seen as an advanced feature in terms of technology development, it also meant that older adults did not make decision about which forms of entertainment were offered by Pepper, but that this decision was made *for* them. This—again—positioned older adults as passive AI users, rather than active contributors to the system.

In terms of "bridging" AI and long-term care, the case of pepper highlights the importance of actively including AI systems in existing care practices and care routines, instead "parachuting in" technology without human support. While older adults found the suggested activities from Pepper engaging and entertaining, the use of Pepper did not necessarily or automatically ease the workload of caregivers. On the contrary, their time and resources were required to facilitate interactions and to assist resident-robot communication:

> *"I can't leave Pepper alone, someone has to be next to it. And that is a problem of manpower."*

It hence became obvious that a full integration of Pepper in long-term care would require additional staff and resources to enable care staff to actively include, and meaningfully engage with pepper on an everyday basis.

The Robot Seal "Paro"

The development of the robotic seal Paro began in 1993 as a form of activation therapy for older adults, often used with people living with dementia [32]. Designed as "socially assistive" [11, p. 84], Paro responds to touch and speech, which makes it a classic example of emotional robotics [17]. Its design—the resemblance of a baby seal—was chosen deliberately, as unfamiliar animals tend to be accepted more easily [33]. Paro's design features include light sensors and touch sensors on its head, whiskers, flippers, back, and belly, a white anti-bacterial coat, as well as its "baby face" with large eyes that open and close [32]. While in Japan, its country of origin, more than 60% of Paro robots are owned by private customers [34], in Europe and the United States Paro is mostly used in public long-term care settings [32].

A scoping review identified three main challenges in the implementation of Paro. The first is its high costs, including acquisition costs of around 6.000€ and costs for training of care staff regarding adequate use of the robot. Second, concerns of infection arise due to the robot being passed between residents and not having removeable/washable fur. Third, research identified a certain stigma of interacting with an animal robot, as some individuals perceive it as "toylike", potentially fostering feelings of infantilization. Also, negative emotional responses, such as fear and anger have been observed, often linked to individuals' past experiences or personal attitudes toward animals [8].

The separation of care and Paro in the ALGOCARE project became apparent with difficulties regarding hygiene, as Paro was hardly used during the peak phase of the corona pandemic, because care staff feared that Paro might cause Covid-19 infections when used by several residents. After the Covid-19 pandemic, care staff started to use Paro regularly again, but efforts were still made to keep residents safe, for instance, through disinfecting the robot regularly. However, this was still seen as not sufficient:

> *"So, you have to make sure the residents' hands are clean, because the fur is almost impossible to clean. [...] Of course, we also work with disinfectant wipes and that's why its fur has turned a bit yellow over time."*

This example highlights that even though Paro was used in a community setting—in groups with a maximum of 12 older adults—it partly separated residents from each other because it could not be used well in a group setting, which would have been desirable in the community context that characterizes many long-term care homes.

However, Paro is also a good example for how AI and care might come together successfully, particularly, through designing technologies in a way that can be easily integrated into the everyday practices of older adults and care staff alike. In the interviews, care staff often highlighted that they would use Paro to engage older residents into dialogues about past experiences. Also, they would provide them information with how the system worked. One care giver explains:

> *"The way I do it with residents is to say: 'Paro isn't real, right? There is a battery in its belly and Paro is able to react because of it. It's a modern device that has sensors built in, so when you touch Paro it moves.' So I explain to residents the technology behind it."*

Although this explanation does not go into great depth, it shows how AI in long-term care can also be an invitation towards residents to build knowledge about how (AI-)technologies work, potentially strengthening digital competencies and inclusion of an often digitally excluded group [6].

Outlook and Conclusions: Pathways Towards AI-Enriched Long-Term Care

The three examples we have discussed in this chapter show that even though there are high hopes that AI will provide the tools necessary to navigate several challenges of long-term care in times of demographic change, there is still much work to be done to meaningfully integrate AI-systems into existing care practices, routines and networks. AI does not automatically make care more efficient, effective or precise, but changes and alters the ways in which care is provided, and the ideals of good care are put into practice. For future research, we propose to explore further how AI can be meaningfully integrated into care systems beyond claims of efficiency and productivity of care. Based on our reflections in this chapter, we propose three pathways for understanding what AI-enriched care might look like.

Pathway 1: Involving Older Adults into AI-Development Practices

First, our data made clear that lack of training data on older adults' activities and everyday practices is a major challenge for AI development in the long-term care sector. Practices of using existing datasets or creating synthetic data, which AI developers turned to as (cheaper) alternatives than collecting real-world data, however, also came with their own challenges: AI developers hardly engaged with the long-term care sector and had little idea about the actual settings they were developing technologies for. This resulted into a troubling separation between AI development and long-term care, where one seemed to lack in-depth knowledge about the other. This might lead to stereotypical assumptions about older adults in technology development, an aspect of ageism that has been studied in-depth by many scholars (e.g [19, 4, 27]).

This highlights the need to actively involve user groups into the development of AI for the long-term care sector. Responsible and participatory innovation strategies [35], that involve stakeholders in innovation practices, have neither been fully developed nor properly contextualized in the LTC sector. While there is a widespread consensus between technology developers, LTC stakeholders and policy makers that AI implementation in LTC needs to involve care workers and older people alike, the potentials of participatory AI design and implementation have been hardly tapped into [36]. To enable the meaningful integration of AI into complex systems of care, there is a need to develop methods of participatory AI-innovation, to ensure that end-users are more effectively integrated into the development as well as the implementation of AI in long-term care.

Pathway 2: Bridging Human and Technological Vulnerability

In the context of long-term care AI technology often is framed as adaptive and supportive, while older adults are framed as passive, un-agentic and in need of support and protection [37]. To some extent, our examples challenged such binary thinking as both—older adults and AI-systems—emerged as vulnerable actors that were in need of (different types of) care. For example, the comparison of Paro to a 'raw egg' (as one carer shares in an interview) suggests the need to manage and protect it. Paro also needed regular care to make sure that his fur was clean and stayed white. This highlights that involving (AI-)technologies in the long-term care sector means acknowledging that technologies need care, too [13]. It is therefore unlikely that AI will ease the staff shortages of the care sector—at least not in the short run. The effective and sustainable establishment of AI-enriched care calls for resources, competences and budgets to link AI and care practices on an everyday basis. These (often invisible) AI-care practices required to make AI-technologies work in everyday life should not overlooked when AI is implemented in the long-term care sector [3].

Pathway 3: Bridging Through Meaningful Connections

Lastly, our examples also showed that older long-term care residents actively engage with AI-technologies and attempt to independently understand their functionality. However, the analysis further indicates that these engagements are rarely acknowledged by other actors involved in the technology development process. Instead, old age is frequently associated with a general disinterest in AI-technologies: "*Older people are, for the most part, creatures of habit; it's difficult to introduce them to new technology.*" Recognising older adults' interest and willingness to interact with technology beyond ageist stereotypes that position them as uninterested and incompetent in relation to new technologies [12] and instead addressing them as agentic actors in the process of data production and technology implementation would not only highlight the diversity of experiences in old age, but also allow older adults to engage with and understand the technologies actually deployed for their own safety and support [7]. This change of perspective, for example by applying participatory approaches, challenges dominant narratives about who is seen as capable of shaping technological futures [9]. This vision for AI-enriched care would also therefore include the acknowledgement of shared learning practices—in older adults, technology developers and care staff—that need to be supported and structured through information and learning opportunities. Through such a shared learning space, AI-enriched care might ultimately become an opportunity to foster a relational dynamic where AI technology and care can mutually and continuously enrich one another.

To summarise, our insights highlight that the integration of AI into long-term care is not simply a matter of technological optimisation but a process that also requires social, material, and ethical considerations. Bridging the gap between human and artificial intelligence means recognising AI not as a solution or replacement for human care but as part of a complex network of care. Only by acknowledging the agency of older adults, the vulnerabilities of both human and technology, and the necessity of participatory development, AI in long-term care can evolve in ways that support existing care practices.

Useful Resources

WHO Policy Brief: Ageism in Artificial Intelligence for Health: https://www.who.int/publications/i/item/9789240040793.

Review Questions

1. Explain the meaning of "techno-solutionism" in the context of long-term care and AI.
2. How does ageism manifest in the development and implementation of AI technologies for long-term care?
3. Name two specific strategies that are proposed to create "bridging" of care and AI?

Answers to Review Questions

1. Techno-solutionism in long-term care and AI refers to the belief that AI-technologies alone can solve complex challenges in care. It assumes that AI will

make care more efficient and effective, without considering the social, ethical, and practical complexities of care.

2. Ageism in AI refers to bias that exclude, disadvantage, or misrepresent older adults. For long-term care it appears in multiple ways: AI systems are often trained on data that excludes older adults, AI developers may hold stereotypes about later life, and needs and perspectives of older adults are often overlooked in AI implementation. This can lead to technologies that are discriminatory or at least inefficient.
3. A central strategy to bridge AI and care is participatory design and its shared learning opportunities. Shared learning spaces, where technology developers, care staff, and older adults exchange knowledge and experiences, can help align AI-technologies with care practices, make AI more inclusive and ensure ethical practices of AI in long-term care.

Funding Katrin Lehner's and Vera Gallistl's work has been funded by the Vienna Science and Technology Fund (WWTF) and by the State of Lower Austria through project ICT20-055 (Grant-ID: 10.47379/ICT20055).

References

1. Chen L-K. Gerontechnology and artificial intelligence: better care for older people. Arch Gerontol Geriatr. 2022;91:104252. https://doi.org/10.1016/j.archger.2020.104252.
2. Chen LK. Artificial intelligence in medicine and healthcare. J Clin Gerontol Geriatrics. 2018;9:77–8.
3. Chevallier M. Staging Paro: the care of making robot(s) care. Soc Stud Sci. 2023;53:635–59.
4. Chu CH, Nyrup R, Leslie K, Shi J, Bianchi A, Lyn A, McNicholl M, Khan S, Rahimi S, Grenier A. Digital ageism: challenges and opportunities in artificial intelligence for older adults. The Gerontologist. 2022;62:947–55. https://doi.org/10.1093/geront/gnab167.
5. Clarke AE. Situationsanalyse: grounded theory nach dem postmodern turn. Springer VS; 2012.
6. Gallistl V, Banday MUL, Berridge C, Grigorovich A, Jarke J, Mannheim I, Marshall B, Martin W, Moreira T, Van Leersum CM, Peine A. Addressing the black box of AI-A model and research agenda on the co-constitution of aging and artificial intelligence. The Gerontologist. 2024;64:gnae039. https://doi.org/10.1093/geront/gnae039.
7. Gallistl V, von Laufenberg R. Caring for data in later life: the datafication of ageing as a matter of care. Inf Commun Soc. 2024;27:774–89. https://doi.org/10.1080/1369118X.2023.2279554.
8. Hung L, Liu C, Woldum E, Au-Yeung A, Berndt A, Wallsworth C, Horne N, Gregorio M, Mann J, Chaudhury H. The benefits of and barriers to using a social robot PARO in care settings: a scoping review. BMC Geriatr. 2019;19:232. https://doi.org/10.1186/s12877-019-1244-6.
9. Jarke J, Manchester H. Datafied ageing futures: regimes of anticipation and participatory futuring. Big Data Soc. 2025;12. https://doi.org/10.1177/20539517241306363.
10. Kim KI, Gollamudi SS, Steinhubl S. Digital technology to enable aging in place. Exp Gerontol. 2017;88:25–31.
11. Kolling T, Haberstroh J, Kapspar R, Pantel J, Oswald F, Knopf M. Evidence and deployment-based research into care for the elderly using emotional robots. GeroPsych. 2013;26:83–8.
12. Köttl H, Gallistl V, Rohner R, Ayalon L. "But at the age of 85? Forget it!": internalized ageism, a barrier to technology use. J Aging Stud. 2021;59:100971. https://doi.org/10.1016/j.jaging.2021.100971.

13. Lipp B. Caring for robots: how care comes to matter in human-machine interfacing. Soc Stud Sci. 2023;53:660–85. https://doi.org/10.1177/03063127221081446.
14. Lukkien DR, Nap HH, Buimer HP, Peine A, Boon WPC, Ket JC, Minkman MMN, Moors EHM. Toward responsible artificial intelligence in long-term care: a scopingreview on practical approaches. The Gerontologist. 2021;63:155–68. https://doi.org/10.1093/geront/gnab180.
15. Manzeschke A, Assadi G, Viehöver W. The role of big data in ambient assisted living. Int Rev Inform Ethics. 2016;24:40–5.
16. Meade R. Bias in machine learning: how facial recognition models show signs of racism, sexism and ageism. Towards Data Science. 2021.
17. Meyer S. Mein Freund der Roboter: Servicerobotik für ältere Menschen; eine Antwort auf den demografischen Wandel? Berlin und Offenbach: VDE-Verlag; 2011.
18. Mishra D, Romero GA, Pande A, Nachenahalli Bhuthegowda B, Chaskopoulos D, Shrestha B. An exploration of the pepper robot's capabilities: unveiling its potential. Appl Sci. 2024;14:110. https://doi.org/10.3390/app14010110.
19. Neves BB, Petersen A, Vered M, Carter A, Omori M. Artificial intelligence in long-term care: technological promise, aging anxieties, and sociotechnical ageism. J Appl Gerontol. 2023;42:1274–82. https://doi.org/10.1177/07334648231157370.
20. Obst L, Bielefeldt F, von der Weth R, Dick M. Service robots in nursing homes (SeRoNu): a holistic model of influencing factors. Gruppe Interaktion Organisation. 2022;53:285–93. https://doi.org/10.1007/s11612-022-00639-4.
21. Peine A, Neven L. The co-constitution of ageing and technology—a model and agenda. Ageing Soc. 2021;41:2845–66. https://doi.org/10.1017/S0144686X20000641.
22. Provenrobotics. Facts about pepper the robot. 2024. Available from: https://provenrobotics.ai/facts-about-pepper-the-robot/. Last access: 6 Feb 2025.
23. PwC. Sherlock in health. 2024. Available from: https://www.pwc.de/de/gesundheitswesen-und-pharma/studie-sherlock-in-health.pdf. Last access: 6 Feb 2025.
24. Rubeis G. The disruptive power of artificial intelligence. Ethical aspects of gerontechnology in elderly care. Arch Gerontol Geriatr. 2020;91:104186. https://doi.org/10.1016/j.archger.2020.104186.
25. Stommel W, de Rijk L, Boumans R. "Pepper, what do you mean?" Miscommunication and repair in robot-led survey interaction. In: 2022 31st IEEE international conference on robot and human interactive communication (RO-MAN). 2022, pp. 385–92. https://doi.org/10.1109/RO-MAN53752.2022.9900528.
26. Stypinska J. Ageism in AI: new forms of age discrimination in the era of algorithms and artificial intelligence. 39. Paper presented at the CAIP, Bologna, Italy. 2021. https://doi.org/10.4108/eai.20-11-2021.2314200.
27. Stypinska J. AI ageism: a critical roadmap for studying age discrimination and exclusion in digitalized societies. AI & Soc. 2023;38:665–77. https://doi.org/10.1007/s00146-022-01553-5.
28. Tanwar R, Nandal N, Zamani M, Manaf AA. Pathway of trends and technologies in fall detection: a systematic review. Healthcare (Basel). 2022;10:172. https://doi.org/10.3390/healthcare10010172.
29. Thakur N, Han CY. A study of fall detection in assisted living: identifying and improving the optimal machine learning method. J Sens Actuator Netw. 2021;10:39. https://doi.org/10.3390/jsan10030039.
30. Wachsmuth I. Robots like me: challenges and ethical issues in aged care. Front Psychol. 2018;9:432. https://doi.org/10.3389/fpsyg.2018.00432.
31. Wang Z, Ramamoorthy V, Gal U, Guez A. Possible life saver: a review on human fall detection technology. Robotics. 2020;9:55. https://doi.org/10.3390/robotics9030055.
32. Pfadenhauer M, Dukat C. Robot caregiver or robot-supported caregiving? The performative deployment of the social robot PARO in dementia care. Int J Soc Robot. 2015;7:393–406. https://doi.org/10.1007/s12369-015-0284-0.
33. Shibata T, Tanie K. Physical and affective interaction between human and mental commit robot. In: Proc. IEEE Int. Conf. Robot. Autom. (ICRA). Seoul: IEEE; 2001.

34. Shibata T. Therapeutic seal robot as biofeedback medical device: qualitative and quantitative evaluations of robot therapy in dementia care. Proc IEEE. 2012;100:2527–38. https://doi.org/10.1109/JPROC.2012.2200559.
35. Urbaniak A. Routledge international handbook of participatory approaches in ageing research. London: Routledge; 2023.
36. Fischer B, Peine A, Östlund B. The importance of user involvement: a systematic review of involving older users in technology design. Gerontologist. 2020;60:e513–23. https://doi.org/10.1093/geront/gnz163.
37. Neves B, Omori M, Petersen A. Artificial intelligence for long-term care in later life. In: Handbook on the sociology of health and medicine. Cheltenham: Edward Elgar Publishing; 2023. p. 488–503. https://doi.org/10.4337/9781839104756.00041.
38. Hartmann KV, Rubeis G, Primc N. Healthy and happy? An ethical investigation of Emotion Recognition and Regulation Technologies (ERR) within Ambient Assisted Living (AAL). Sci Eng Ethics. 2024;30:2–2. https://doi.org/10.1007/s11948-024-00470-8.
39. Rubeis G. Adiaphorisation and the digital nursing gaze: liquid surveillance in long-term care. Nurs Philos. 2023;24:e12388. https://doi.org/10.1111/nup.12388.
40. Morozov E. To save everything, click here: the folly of technological solutionism. New York: PublicAffairs; 2013.

Chapter 8
Generative AI to Assist Physicians

Geoffrey Rutledge

Learning Objectives
- To understand the many ways generative AI can assist physicians
- To review the state of the art for generative AI in healthcare
- To develop a rationale for future applications of generative AI in healthcare

Key Terms
- Artificial Intelligence
- Generative AI
- Large language models (LLMs)
- Generative pre-trained transformers
- GPT-4
- Differential diagnoses
- Clinical decision support
- ICD10 diagnostic codes

Summary
The advent of generative AI and large language models (LLMs) has created remarkable opportunities to improve the efficiency and effectiveness of healthcare. So far, generative AI has proven helpful for a variety of administrative, clerical and data-summarization tasks. AI is also very good at making accurate clinical diagnoses when complete patient data (case presentations) are available. AI is able to interview patients and collect basic information but is unable to duplicate the essential role that doctors play. AI offers the opportunity to support and enhance what doctors do, but for the foreseeable future, AI will not be ready to replace doctors.

G. Rutledge (✉)
HealthTap, Sunnyvale, CA, USA
e-mail: geoff@healthtap.com

U. H. Hübner et al. (eds.), *Bridging Artificial and Human Intelligence*, Health Informatics, https://doi.org/10.1007/978-3-032-11938-4_8

Introduction

The advent of generative AI and large language models (LLMs) has transformed our understanding of the capabilities of AI, and has created remarkable opportunities to improve the efficiency and effectiveness of healthcare.

Before the advent of generative AI and LLMs, AI applications relied on diverse methods, from production rule-based expert systems, to probabilistic assessments and Bayesian networks, to data-driven analytic techniques from machine learning. All of these prior AI methods suffer from the same limitation that their ability to respond to a patient scenario was limited. Particularly the rule-based systems suffered a "cliff effect" when confronted with anything that was not explicitly included in their knowledge representation, and they lacked the ability to understand everyday issues that we think of as "common sense."

For this discussion, we are focusing exclusively on AI applications that use generative methods based on LLMs.

The largest LLMs now include such a vast array of information that they can respond appropriately to a much wider range and type of inputs—virtually any human expression. Their performance degrades gracefully at the limit of their encoded knowledge—but when at that limit of knowledge, they are more likely to "hallucinate", or fill in the gaps of knowledge with a reasonable-sounding output for which there is no direct support—LLMs can "make stuff up" [1].

There are many application areas for AI in healthcare [2], as shown in Fig. 8.1. In this chapter, we focus on Clinical Documentation and Workflow automation. We briefly discuss administrative processes and communications, then focus on how AI can help support the workflow of direct clinical care, including automated clinical assessments, documentation, and diagnostic decision support.

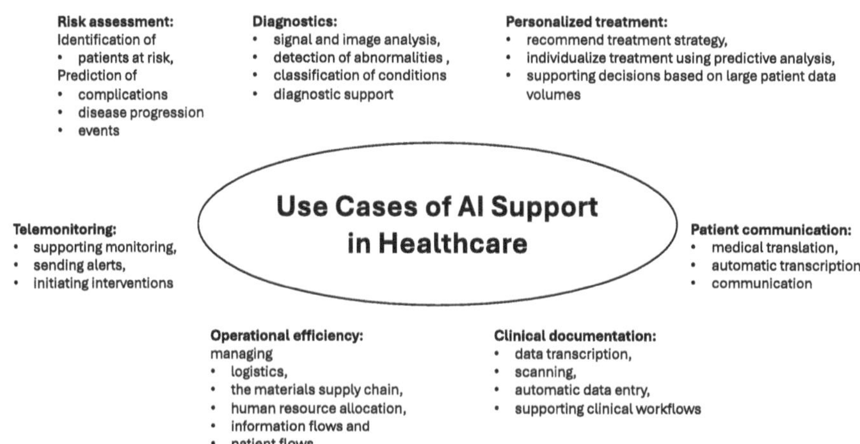

Fig. 8.1 Use cases of AI support in healthcare

Foundation Model LLMs Versus Medical LLMs

LLMs have the ability to respond to virtually any human expression. The largest of the LLMs are so-called "foundation models" that have trillions of parameters that were trained on comprehensive collections of essentially all available electronic documents that represent the bulk of human knowledge, including knowledge of medicine.

Examples of foundation-model LLMs as of early 2025 include Anthropic Claude, OpenAI GPT, Google Gemini, Meta LLaMA, and Mistral. The performance of these foundation model LLMs on medical problems is surprisingly good, even though they were not trained specifically on curated medical data. Perhaps more important than the potential limitations of the scope and accuracy of their training data, is that they suffer to varying degrees from "hallucinations".

The hallucinations that come from generative AI occur in areas where there are no data to offer the correct information; in other words, "hallucinations" occur when there are gaps in knowledge. This has a parallel in human behavior. People who suffer from retrograde amnesia (loss of previous memories) will "make things up" to fill in gaps in their memory, as typically happens in Korsakoff syndrome. People who suffer from Korsakoff syndrome often are unaware that they are making things up. This is called confabulation [3].

Efforts to improve the scope of the medical knowledge of foundation models have focused on refining base models with training on additional more highly curated sources of reliable medical information. The nature of medical applications also demands that the rate of confabulation be minimal, so much effort is directed at measuring and minimizing the rate of confabulation of these models.

Examples of medically trained LLMs include Google Med-PaLM, which is tuned for medical reasoning and Q&A. Nuance DAX Copilot and AWS Healthscribe are focused on medical scribing to generate notes in the EHR. Hippocratic AI is focused on medical conversations. Clinical Camel is an experimental medical LLM built as an open-sourced project on LLaMa.

Medical LLMs that are tailored to a specific clinical task may be less performant on tasks that involve interpreting what people say during a medical interview, because the foundation model underlying the medical LLM is smaller.

Administrative Simplification

Claims Coding

AI applications are already available that support insurance billing and claims management. For example, Fathom (fathom.com) and Nym Health (nym.health) both offer applications that use clinical language understanding to fully automate generation of Current Procedural Terminology/Healthcare Common Procedure Coding

System (CPT / HCPCS) procedure codes, and verify that the International Classification of diseases-10th ed. (ICD10) diagnostic codes support the selected procedure codes.

These tools operate "behind the scenes" and out of sight of patients who receive care. They promise improvements in administrative efficiency and rate of collections, which supports the financial health of a practice—without having an impact on how or what care is delivered.

Applications that restrict their focus to a defined task may achieve better performance with an LLM that is specifically trained for the task at hand. For example, a claims-coding application is trained specifically on the features of a structured coding system (such as CPT and ICD-10). Smaller and open-source foundation models allow incremental training on such information to create a LLM that both responds to unstructured text and identifies the most appropriate and applicable billing codes.

Managing Message Queues

A large opportunity exists for healthcare practices to improve their communications by automating the triage and responses to messages from patients. Whether a message is received by voice on an answering machine, or by text in email, or by a faxed document, AI can interpret and respond to each message with a triage decision and a response or draft of a response for a clinician to review.

Messages regarding scheduling requests or billing concerns are triaged to clerical personnel. Messages of a clinical nature are triaged to a clinician for review, and if a message suggests a more urgent response is needed, it can be flagged and forwarded as needed for attention.

A study from Stanford evaluated the ability of AI to triage patient messages and then draft text responses for the clinicians. They used Epic's MyChart with an integration of GPT-3.5 Turbo for triage (to one of general, results, medications, and paperwork), and GPT-4 to generate the draft message responses [4].

This study found that the draft response was used 20% of the time, but on average, did not reduce the time required by the doctors and nurses to generate the responses. The overall evaluation by the clinicians was positive, with many saying that the draft responses reduced the cognitive effort to craft a response in patient-friendly language, and others commenting that the AI-generated responses were more detailed and lengthy than what they usually would write. However, the reactions from clinicians were heterogeneous, and some thought the AI-generated responses were too lengthy or contained irrelevant information.

One observation from the results of this study is that successful implementation of AI-generated responses to patient messages may benefit from fine tuning how the AI responds to match the desired response characteristics for each clinician.

Clinical Documentation

Chart Review and Summarization

Administrative applications improve operational efficiency, but they do not directly affect or improve the care that is delivered. Because LLMs now embed a deep level of medical knowledge, they can support complex clinical operations: LLMs can process large amounts of structured and unstructured data in a patient's clinical record to help clinicians understand and learn from a patient's past medical history.

A thorough, concise and readable summary of a patient's history is essential for doctors to evaluate and manage their patients (especially new patients). Unfortunately, the volume of previous medical records on a single patient can be overwhelming. A thorough review of a single patient's past records could take many more hours of effort than is available for a doctor to spend. As a result, far too often, a doctor may not be aware of relevant features of a patient's past history that would influence their care.

A recent formal study of AI-generated versus clinician summaries of prior medical records showed a similar rating of the quality of the summaries, but also noted that "AI-authored summaries were less likely to omit important information and more likely to use patient-friendly language" [5].

Another study compared the quality and completeness of AI-generated summaries and treatment recommendations based on the prior medical records for patients with breast cancer. They found that both the AI-generated and the AI-assisted summaries were better than the human summaries. The human summaries required 26 minutes of effort, versus just 1.7 minutes for the AI-generated summaries [6].

Ambient Listening

AI is now being systematically deployed to assist in *generating* original documentation of the clinical encounter. "Ambient listening" applications operate by recording and processing the audio of the doctor-patient encounter to extract the relevant clinical features in the answers to the interviewer's questions. The AI then generates a clinical note that documents the subjective history. The doctor can also dictate as they examine the patient, so that the AI can also fill out the observed clinical findings in the objective section of the encounter note.

Examples of commercially available ambient listening applications include Abridge AI, Augmedix, Robin Healthcare, and IKS Health.

Many health systems are implementing ambient listening medical scribes as their first use of AI in the clinical workflow. Initial evaluations reveal improvements in the ease of documentation, as reported by clinicians, and significant reductions in the need for after-hours time to complete documentation (reduced "pajama time" for the doctors). Doctors also report that having an AI scribe generate the note significantly reduces the cognitive effort required to complete the documentation.

Concerns raised about AI scribes include the possibility that the AI will misinterpret or not understand specific medical terms or complex medical language: They may omit critical details and fail to capture key clinical findings. Perhaps a larger concern is the possibility that the doctors will come to rely on the AI-generated notes without reviewing their details to identify such gaps.

Further studies are needed to confirm the performance of these tools. They require a very high rate of note completeness and accuracy, and a very low rate of hallucinations [7].

Differential Diagnosis

AI solutions that support clinical documentation perform the act of summarizing, organizing, and restating clinical information. They use embedded knowledge to interpret the documentation of findings, diagnoses, tests, and treatments.

There is another and perhaps more exciting application of LLMs in healthcare. The largest of the LLMs have sufficient embedded medical knowledge that they can independently review a set of findings (as enumerated in the clinical documentation) and suggest likely medical diagnoses based on those findings. Studies of the diagnostic capabilities of LLMs have shown remarkable aptitude, with diagnostic performance that is consistently better than that of experts [8].

In a recent study, GPT-4 demonstrated 96% accuracy in diagnosing common ambulatory care cases (versus 72% for doctors), and outperformed the best experts in identifying likely diagnoses in highly complex cases. GPT-4 included the correct diagnosis in its top 10 differential list for 61% of cases, versus medical residents who were correct in 44% of cases, and medical faculty who were correct in 49% [9].

Note that these studies were carried out with foundation LLM models (such as GPT-4) that were not specifically trained on or fine-tuned for medical applications. Multiple medical LLMs under development promise to improve the performance of the foundation models. However, these have so far not demonstrated significantly better diagnostic performance. It remains to be seen if the advances in medical LLMs will occur faster than the advances in performance of the largest of the general purpose LLMs. It may be that for highly specialized tasks in selected domains, a specifically trained LLM will be needed. It does seem clear that for interpreting the meaning of dialog with patients, the general purpose LLMs are exceptionally capable.

Will AI Replace Doctors?

Given the remarkable diagnostic abilities of the LLMs, it is natural to ask if AI is now better than doctors at taking a history and making the diagnosis. It turns out, however, that as of yet, the LLMs fall short for this task. When we ask LLMs to "take the history" by interacting directly with a patient, they fail to identify all the relevant features, and without a complete set of patient features, their diagnostic performance drops [10].

If LLMs are so good at recognizing the diagnosis when they are shown the features, why are they not asking all the right questions to identify those features? It turns out that to select all the right questions requires a level of planning that LLMs are not currently capable of. Physicians know how to think through and systematically pursue structured areas of potential concern. Doctors plan a sequence of questions or inquiries that successively address each area, starting with the most general questions that identify if an area of concern warrants further inquiry.

For example, in thinking through what might be the explanation for a patient's presenting symptoms, a doctor may consider in sequence all the various diagnoses that correspond to congenital, inflammatory, toxic, traumatic, neoplastic, and degenerative etiologies. When a general question in a category suggests it, the doctor pursues that category in more detail. This type of structured or systematic approach to taking the interview is not currently embedded in LLMs.

Without such planning abilities, LLMs typically ask about features that may be present in the most likely explanations for a given patient scenario.

We can imagine that soon it will be possible for an LLM to implement a more structured approach to obtaining a complete and relevant history. However, identifying the relevant differential diagnosis is just the first step of patient care. The next steps require planning and consideration of what testing or treatment approach is best for a patient.

Some of the considerations for planning a testing or treatment strategy include:

- Should the doctor order a confirmatory test for the most likely diagnosis? Or perhaps order tests to exclude the less likely diagnoses?
- Based on the consequences of each potential diagnosis, is it better simply to observe the patient, expecting the problem to resolve on its own? Or perhaps it would be best to recommend a therapeutic trial of a treatment for the likely diagnosis.
- Will the cost of the testing or treatment plan be a barrier to the patient's ability to follow the recommendations?
- Each possible recommendation will depend also on the preferences of the patient, who may have a strong preference for one or another treatment or testing option.

Doctors must in the end identify and communicate the testing and treatment recommendation that is optimal for a patient.

And none of the above mechanistic approaches to diagnosis and treatment planning recognizes the very human need that people have for comfort and support in times of illness, and for confidence that the care they are receiving is the best possible choice for them.

The current state of LLMs is encouraging for the near-term achievement of the first of these steps. The remaining steps will require substantial progress from where we are today. So AI is not yet ready to replace the doctor.

However, there is an important role that AI can play to support rather than replace the physician. The depth of medical knowledge and interpretation capabilities of LLM-based generative AI solutions can provide powerful support for doctors when it is integrated appropriately in the doctors' workflow, and with an understanding of its weaknesses and limitations.

For example, AI can operate in a supervisory capacity to identify gaps in care and suggest actions to close them. It can suggest alternative diagnoses based on features in the chart, perhaps doing so in the background to offer suggestions at the most useful time in the workflow of the doctor's care. Doctors can turn to AI to ask about challenging cases or concerns and receive answers that may expand their differential diagnosis or give them additional ideas for how to test or treat.

An AI-Based Physician Assistant

One powerful application of AI in the everyday workflow of patient care is the virtual physician assistant. In this role, an AI agent can interact directly with a patient seeking care from a doctor by asking the questions that the doctor would ask, and then the AI can write a summary of the patient's answers as a draft clinical note for the doctor.

This type of virtual physician assistant was implemented and has been live in the virtual primary care clinic on HealthTap. The service, which is known as "Dr. A.I.", encourages people who have scheduled an appointment for a video visit with their doctor to engage in a pre-visit interview. The AI is prompted to ask the questions that the doctor would ask, based on the known features of the patient and their reason for the visit. Dr. A.I. implements GPT-4 via API, which allows for setting the patient context, interpreting the patient's answers, and generating the draft clinical note for the doctor.

Importantly, the AI does not offer the patient any diagnoses or treatment plans. At each step, it asks the next question in light of all the previous answers and all other information. The AI asks questions until it sees no more value in asking additional questions, or a fixed question limit is reached, or until the patient asks to end the interview.

After the interview, Dr. A.I. creates a draft clinical note that the doctor reviews at the beginning of the visit. By reviewing the answers to all the questions asked by Dr. A.I., the doctor saves the time it would take them to ask those questions. The doctor also saves time writing their clinical note when they include or build on the draft of the note suggested by Dr. A.I.

Dr. A.I. builds a differential diagnosis for the patient, and asks questions that refine or confirm the diagnoses. It stores a computed differential diagnosis, but does not show that differential to the doctor.

Interestingly, one of the effects of showing the answers to the questions that Dr. A.I. asked is that the doctor may infer the diagnoses that Dr. A.I. was pursuing. The answers remind the doctors of many possible conditions that could explain the patient's symptoms. But the doctor's final diagnosis is not prompted by seeing the list of diagnoses from Dr. A.I.

Evaluation

Evaluating the quality of a medical history can be challenging, because there is no gold standard for what questions should be asked in any given patient scenario. However, because Dr. A.I. records its diagnoses, we can compare the diagnoses that the doctor made (as recorded by the doctor's selection of ICD-10 diagnosis codes) with the differential diagnoses recorded by Dr. A.I.

Table 8.1 shows the results of this evaluation. Because the doctors often code more than one diagnosis at each visit, we record how often each of the doctors' diagnoses was present on the list of Top10 diagnoses generated by Dr. A.I.

In this study, the doctor's first ICD10 diagnosis was found on Dr. A.I.'s differential list in 88% of cases! Interestingly, when the doctor assigned multiple diagnoses to a patient, the subsequent diagnoses were also found on the differential: the second ICD10 diagnosis was found in 80% of cases, and when a third or more diagnoses were coded, those additional diagnoses were found 46% of the time on Dr. A.I's differential list.

The conclusion is that questions asked and the diagnoses generated by a GPT-4 based patient interview correspond to a high degree to the diagnoses assessed by doctors who evaluated the patients. This study shows that it is possible to use generative AI based on the largest foundation models to engage patients in a medically relevant dialog that identifies the likely causes of a patient's medical symptoms [11].

Table 8.1 Doctors' ICD10 versus Dr. A.I. diagnoses

	Top10 Dr. A.I.	Top3 Dr. A.I.	Top1 Dr. A.I.
1st ICD10	88% (109/124)	81% (100/124)	62% (77/124)
2nd ICD10	80% (45/56)	61% (34/56)	23% (13/56)
3rd–7th ICD10	46% (25/55)	27% (15/55)	4% (2/55)

Outlook and Conclusions

Although the current state of AI is incredibly promising, we should not forget that:

> For the foreseeable future, GPT-4 cannot be used in medical settings without direct human supervision. [12]

The recent development of generative AI built upon LLMs has created fantastic opportunities to improve the effectiveness and efficiency of many clinical operations. We are already seeing rapid adoption of administrative, clinical summarization, and ambient listening applications. We are also seeing early efforts to leverage the clinical knowledge of LLMs to support and improve more complex medical decision making tasks.

The further refinement of medical LLMs, and the rapid pace of improvement of the foundation model LLMs both promise to make future applications of AI within the clinical workflow even more powerful.

Useful Resources

1. ChatGPT, MD: How AI-Empowered Patients & Doctors Can Take Back Control of American Medicine, by Robert Pearl MD, 297 pp., Apr 9, 2024
2. Coursera—AI in Healthcare Specializations
    - Offers courses from top universities like Stanford and Johns Hopkins
    - Key courses:
        - "AI in Healthcare" by Stanford University
        - "Machine Learning for Healthcare" by Stanford
3. Journals to follow
    - NPJ Digital Medicine (Nature Partner Journal Digital Medicine)
    - JMIR Medical Informatics (Journal of Medical Internet Research
    - Artificial Intelligence in Medicine
    - Nature Digital Medicine
    - NEJM AI (New England Journal of Medicine Artificial Intelligence)
    - JAMIA (Journal of American Medical Informatics Association)

Review Questions

1. What does GPT mean?
2. When a complete case description is available, which is better at making the diagnosis: Expert doctors or generative AI based on the largest foundation models?
3. Will AI soon replace doctors?
4. What are the impediments to an AI replacing the doctor?

Answers to Review Questions

1. Generative Pre-trained Transformer
2. Generative AI, in particular GPT-4o and above outperform doctors only if all the important features are known and included in the inputs.

3. No. Not soon. But AI can support doctors now, and that support is becoming increasingly more valuable. Eventually it is likely AI will replace many basic functions that doctors do—but that time remains a long way off.
4. The main issue today is that generative AI does not have the ability to plan—to look ahead at the myriad of possible future outcomes for any / all choices of action (observation, test, treat). But even when that capability is added, AI will still need to learn how to understand a patient's individual preferences that affect their optimal choice, and their willingness to follow recommendations. Finally, to replace the doctors, AI would need to offer empathetic and compassionate support for people who are in physical or mental distress as a result of their health.

References

1. Kim Y, Jeong H, Chen S, et al. Medical hallucination in foundation models and their impact on healthcare. 2025. https://doi.org/10.1101/2025.02.28.25323115. Available from https://arxiv.org/abs/2503.05777. Last access: 23 Mar 2025.
2. Genovese A. The potential applications of artificial intelligence in healthcare. 2025. Created in BioRender https://BioRender.com/g74f622.
3. Korsakoff Syndrome. Wikipedia. Available from https://en.wikipedia.org/wiki/Korsakoff_syndrome. Last access: 23 Mar 2025.
4. Garcia P, Ma S, Shah S, et al. Artificial intelligence–generated draft replies to patient inbox messages. JAMA Netw Open. 2024;7(3):e243201. https://doi.org/10.1001/jamanetworkopen.2024.3201.
5. Shemtob L, Nouri A, Sullivan A, et al. Comparing AI – versus clinician-authored summaries of simulated primary care electronic health records. medRxiv. 2025. https://doi.org/10.1101/2025.02.21.25322674.
6. Chen P, Jung J, Kim Y, et al. AI-assisted clinical summary and treatment planning for cancer care: a comparative study of human vs. AI-based approaches. J Clin Oncol. 2024;42(16 suppl):1523. https://doi.org/10.1200/JCO.2024.42.16_suppl.1523.
7. Lee C, Britto S, Diwan K. Evaluating the impact of artificial intelligence (AI) on clinical documentation efficiency and accuracy across clinical settings: a scoping review. Cureus. 2024;16(11):e73994. https://doi.org/10.7759/cureus.73994.
8. Erikson A, Möller S, Ryg J. Use of GPT-4 to diagnose complex clinical cases. NEJM AI. 2024;1(1). https://doi.org/10.1056/AIp2300031.
9. Rutledge GW. Diagnostic accuracy of GPT-4 on common clinical scenarios and challenging cases. Learn Health Syst. 2024;8:e10438. https://doi.org/10.1002/lrh2.10438.
10. Hager P, Jungmann F, Holland R, et al. Evaluation and mitigation of the limitations of large language models in clinical decision-making. Nat Med. 2024;30(9):2613–22. https://doi.org/10.1038/s41591-024-03097-1.
11. Rutledge G. A generative AI-based virtual physician assistant AAAI spring symposium series. Available from: https://ojs.aaai.org/index.php/AAAI-SS/article/view/31182/33342. Last access: 23 Mar 2025.
12. Lee P, Goldberg C, Kohanne I. The AI revolution in medicine: GPT-4 and beyond. London: Pearson Education, Inc; 2023.

Chapter 9
AI Supporting Nursing Documentation, Workflows and Patient Care

Evelyn J. S. Hovenga

Learning Objectives
- To understand functional capabilities of AI technologies
- To understand the necessary data and technical ecosystem fundamental requirements for trustworthy and beneficial AI use
- To consider making use of AI to support nursing documentation, and workflow
- To assess potential value of making use of robots
- To apply agreed ethical principles when making use of AI
- To explain risk mitigation strategies to be considered prior to AI use
- To identify nursing practice components likely to benefit from AI support

Key Terms
- Artificial Intelligence (AI)
- AI functional hierarchy
- Robots
- Nursing workflow
- Nursing Documentation
- Decision Support
- Data concepts
- Interoperability
- Patient care
- Ethics
- Risk mitigation

E. J. S. Hovenga (✉)
Faculty of Health Sciences, Australian Catholic University, Melbourne, VIC, Australia

U. H. Hübner et al. (eds.), *Bridging Artificial and Human Intelligence*, Health Informatics, https://doi.org/10.1007/978-3-032-11938-4_9

Summary
This chapter covers some of the fundamental functionalities of various AI technologies. The importance of data quality and interoperability is identified and need to be considered as pre-requisites to the safe, efficient and effective use of AI technologies. These concepts are described in terms of known relationships between data, information, knowledge and information system technologies within any digital health ecosystem. Risk mitigation strategies to be considered prior to AI adoption to support nursing practice at any point of care need to be explored. It is argued that AI adoption, including the use of robots, has the potential to reduce nursing time spent on documentation and workflow inefficiencies. The chapter concludes with a discussion about patient care and ethical considerations associated with the use of AI technologies.

Introduction: Artificial Intelligence and Nursing Practice

Artificial intelligence (AI)'s evolution began at the same time as computing technologies evolved. These technical and scientific advances have influenced the health industry generally and may be applicable to any of its knowledge domains, including nursing practice. AI technologies most commonly relate to any aspect of data and information processing. The latter is a core function used by nurses and midwives to support their practice, so let's explore how AI can best support nursing practice and enable nurses and midwives to have a positive impact on population health.

As a rule, AI needs to make use of big, accurate, complete and unbiased data to provide meaningful results. One needs to appreciate the relationships between data characteristics, computing processing capabilities and data exchange schema in use, in order to acquire an understanding of how AI can best support nursing practice. These data, information and communication technological relationships determine the quality of data used by AI technologies.

We have an international need for extensive collaboration within the nursing (including midwifery) profession and with all relevant stakeholders, to influence useful development of AI technologies. Such collaboration also requires us to ensure that nursing's documentation can be used as source data for a variety of AI applications. Such capacity can best be achieved by adopting the use of a global standard language and data structures for point of care data, collected by nurses and midwives within a suitably defined digital health ecosystem to generate large high quality datasets needed for the use of AI applications to support:

- patient safety;
- nursing workflows;
- the demonstration of the value of nurses and midwives' contribution to health care;
- developing decision support algorithms and artificial intelligence protocols;

- the management of nursing resources;
- data analytics making use of quality coded nursing data;
- continuity of care across health services;
- enhancing patient outcomes within and between health services; and facilitate:
- cross-organization research;
- meaningful interoperability;
- inter-professional documentation;
- data driven decision making at all levels within the health system;
- generation of nursing knowledge and wisdom across the continuum of health and health care;
- support for population health and nursing practice;
- person-centred outcomes measurement;

This chapter explores these relationships and examines if and how these AI technologies can best support nursing (and midwifery) practice. First the technologies that need to be considered are identified and described. We then explore their functionalities in terms of:

1. an AI functional hierarchy based on complexity,
2. nursing practice relationships and
3. current working environments.

An Important AI Pre-requisite: Quality Data

AI support for nursing documentation, workflows and patient care generally is largely dependent upon the quality of data available and used for the development and use of AI technologies. Data quality is a critical pre-cursor. Data quality characteristics include accuracy, consistency, validity, timeliness, accessibility, reliability, completeness, uniqueness and comprehensiveness. In order to generate large data sets as required for the effective use of AI technologies, there needs to be system interoperability, a complex concept dependent upon system compliance with an agreed set of technical standards.

This author advocates the use of the ISO standard categorical structure [1, 2] to represent nursing practice in terminological systems. These categories can be linked to any standard nursing terminology (SNT). They essentially provide a nursing information model compliant with the nursing process. Their adoption enables these concepts to relate to clinical knowledge models (archetypes) structured in accordance with the ISO 13606-2: 2019 standard [3] as adopted within next generation electronic health record (EHR) systems. Each model's attributes can then be bound to SNTs and used as standard nursing data value sets as shown in Fig. 9.1. This image reflects the critical data and technical infrastructure relationship that optimises semantic interoperability as explained later.

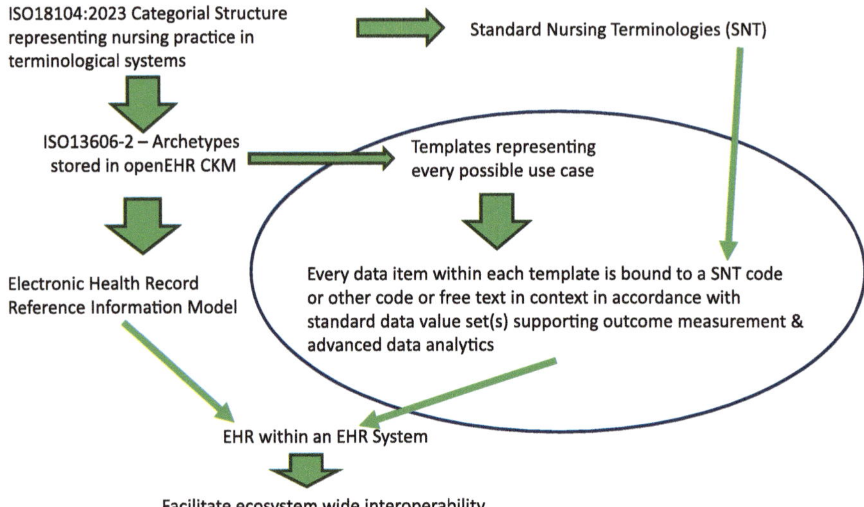

Fig. 9.1 Critical AI pre-requisites, data quality and interoperability

AI Sciences and Technologies

AI sciences and technologies are commonly described using the following terms (Table 9.1).

Each of these technologies has its own focus such as, data characteristics, data relationships, types of data and/or specific computing processing capabilities. All of these technologies need to make use of data originally generated somewhere at a point in time, known as 'source data'. These data need to be representative of a knowledge domain or a population of interest and be computable at the back end of a computer system by complying with agreed standard formats. Computability is determined by access to atomic level data elements (data points) which can be analysed and processed by a computer.

There is a hierarchy of AI capabilities as described by Peter and Riemer [4]. This hierarchy essentially represents the AI technology development pathway. These authors developed what they called a 'capabilities stack' used to explain the broad range of capabilities that AI has to offer ranging from least to most complexity. Their 'stack' consists of seven basic kinds of capability. It starts with the:

1. **Recognition of patterns of data** associated with images, text or sound.
2. These patterns can then be **classified into distinct categories,** such as healthcare classifications, terminologies or ontologies.
3. AI can be used to **predict future outcomes,** for example by assessing patient risk based on historical patterns,
4. From which **recommendations** regarding the most suitable option from a set of alternatives can be made. See example in Box 9.1.

Table 9.1 Terms of AI sciences and technologies

Technologies	Descriptions
Data science, taxonomies and ontologies	Represents a multidisciplinary approach combining principles and practices from the fields of mathematics, statistics, computer engineering and AI.
Data analytics	A component of the data sciences. Analytical accuracy is dependent upon the quality of data accessed and used by humans or technologies.
Natural language processing	The application of computational techniques adopted to analyse and synthesize our documentation and speech. The latter is used for voice recognition.
Biometrics	Body measurements and recognition of people's unique physical and behavioural characteristics.
Neural networks	A type of machine learning that uses a model inspired by biological neural networks to teach computers to process data. The modelling focus is on relationships between dependent and independent variables representing knowledge domains often in the form of domain ontologies.
Robotics	Represents a multidisciplinary approach consisting of mathematics, computer science and engineering to design, construct, program, operate and use robots to replicate, substitute or assist humans to complete tasks of various complexity. They have been in use, predominantly by the manufacturing industry, since the 1960s. Robots vary in terms of their ability to perform complex tasks. Their development is a growing industry providing endless applications and possibilities for their use in the health industry.

Box 9.1 Example of Recommendations Made Based on Historical Data

For example, when a nurse documents a patient's assessment results, the system can provide historical data on the number of past patients with similar nursing diagnoses, the interventions that were implemented, and the outcomes achieved for each intervention. This allows the system to generate best practice recommendations for the most appropriate intervention for the current patient. These recommendations can also be tailored to the individual's past behaviors, preferences, and dislikes, thereby supporting a more personalized and person-centered approach to care.

Note: to enable this capability nurses need to make use of a standard nursing terminology (at the back end of the system) and the record management system (EHR) in use needs to be compliant with the ISO 18104 standard [1] which describes the categorial structure for the representation of nursing practice in terminological systems.

5. The next AI capability is **automation** which builds on predictive capabilities. For example, a device that monitors blood sugar levels (content) and automates the administration of insulin (controlled use).
6. Then with greater complexity AI is able to **generate original content** by mimicking characteristics of its training data, such as text, images, video or sound.

One common example is the now widespread use of Chat GPT or similar AI technologies that enable changes to be made to text, images or video clips.
7. The most complex capability is where AI facilitates **user interactions** such as via the use of chatbots or life-like avatars. This leverages machine learning and natural language processing and more, to understand users and real-time context to drive meaningful interactions, including the use of robots to generate train tickets for example.

A robot is defined by ISO as a 'programmed actuated mechanism with a degree of autonomy to perform locomotion, manipulation or positioning'. A robot includes the control system. Examples of a mechanical structure of robots are manipulator, mobile platform and wearable robot. A robot controller is a set of hardware and software components implementing logic and power control, and other functions which allow monitoring and controlling of the behaviour of a robot and its interaction and communication with other objects and humans in the environment [5].

Robotic applications may be used to address critical challenges in nursing and midwifery. With increasing demands for healthcare services and a shortage of skilled workers, robotics offers solutions that enhance efficiency, safety, and patient care. From assisting nurses in routine tasks, to providing emotional support in elder care, robots have the potential to revolutionise these fields. However, their adoption also introduces risks that require careful management.

Each of these AI capabilities can also have negative impacts. Scanning big existing data to distinguish and segment data based on common elements or other set criteria may result in biased or inaccurate results if the data used was not representative of the domain as a whole. There is also the risk of generating 'group think' recommendations based on frequent use of certain concepts, for example the notion of 'we've always done it this way', which prevents innovation or impedes transformative behaviours. Generative AI risks the production of deepfakes, digitally modified images or videos no longer representing world reality.

Use of AI Technologies and Risk Mitigation

All of the above AI capabilities demonstrate the inter-dependencies between source data, the data supply chain and computing capability. When considering the use of AI in the health industry it is imperative that we understand the potential impact of how data and computing technologies are managed. Computer processing is at its best when data are standardized at the back end. This requires us to be cognizant of the data supply chain in terms of where and by whom are data collected, where and by which technologies are these data further processed, transferred, linked and shared to where data are discarded or stored and retrievable for further use. Ideally digital health datasets are in place to support the testing, use and evaluation of AI in nursing and midwifery [6].

Big data is used by AI technologies for further data processing, including data analytics. Clinical data is aggregated and processed to, for example, determine best practice, monitor outcomes, for public health purposes or to report health system performance. Data sharing between systems for any purpose is dependent upon system interoperability as well as the use of federated clinical data repositories (CDR) able to operate in a coordinated fashion. The latter may be achieved by a central CDR able to orchestrate the others.

Data needs to be labelled or standardized to optimize computer processing capabilities. When transferred between systems the receiving system needs to be able to interpret and compute the data in a manner that does not lose its original meaning (semantics). Data needs to be saved in a non-volatile storage system so that the data's value can be reliably retrieved at any time. Different health data exchange schema are in use. Each of these makes use of an adopted data interchange standard. The ability to adopt any given standard is dependent upon each system's architecture or platform in use.

The data transferred via any interchange schema ideally has the highest possible level of expressivity, that is the ability to communicate the key concepts/ideas in a contextual computable form. This requires the adoption of evidence based models/artifacts to represent concepts as described in the ISO 13606 Part 2 standard [3] based on the openEHR International standard specifications [7, 8]. These artifacts can also be made use of by the Health Level Seven (HL7) Fast Health Interoperability Resources (FHIR) standard [9]. Many countries and/or other entities have adopted their own Health Information Exchange (HIE) protocols [10] in an effort to make the best possible use of legacy systems built on proprietary architectures in the absence of an open standard platform. There is an urgent need to optimize EHRs in a manner that supports AI applications [11]. Next generation EHRs are designed to meet this need.

Legacy systems consist of outdated hardware, software, file formats or programming languages still in use. Such systems are often critically supporting day to day operational activities. New systems need to be compatible with old systems and data formats, this makes system updates challenging. The continuing use of legacy systems results in a technology debt representing a cost of future reworking required to fix issues caused by short term solutions that prioritize expedience over long term design. One could argue that the adoption of HIE protocols are a short term fix that prevents the optimum use of new AI technologies. Similarly, the continuing non-use of a standard nursing terminology (SNT) or inability of legacy systems to use SNTs, prevents the nursing profession from demonstrating the value of services provided or to make good use of AI technologies.

Foundational Data Concepts and Interoperability

Data are 're-interpretable representations of information in a formalized manner suitable for communication, interpretation or processing by human beings or by automatic means' [12]. Data elements represent descriptors of things, concepts or codes, such as age at admission or eye colour or phone number or an international classification of diseases (ICD) code. Data elements make up data sets representing any knowledge domain. Data elements are used to standardize agreed meaning and acceptable representation of data use within a defined context. Data elements may be identified to represent any level of detail from the atomic to the most general level of granularity [13]. For example, Table 9.2 shows the difference between data and data elements that provide context.

There is no need for nurses to understand these technical aspects in any detail. It is extremely useful to just have a sound understanding of the differences between electronic data structures and their data accessibility and retrievability. Data access and use with meaning began with the introduction of relational databases. These were designed to represent entity relationships where each entity had the same key data element that enabled linkage. Such connections then enabled electronic transactions between databases to occur. The next level of complexity made use of 'objects' that represent any concept by incorporating context to provide meaning. From a data management perspective ISO [12] refers to such objects as 'data models', a graphical, lexical or combined representation of data specifying their properties, structure and interrelationships. Archetypes represent such object models. From a general information systems perspective these are also known as 'constraint models'.

Today interoperability is achieved by making use of Health Level Seven (HL7)'s Fast Healthcare Interoperability Resources (FHIR) [9], openEHR's archetypes [8] and/or the Observational Medical Outcomes Partnership (OMOP) Common Data Model (CDM) [14]. The use of data models (objects) was followed by the use of 'agents' which incorporate not only such context but also actions or interactive processes. Agents represent the highest level of complexity and can be modeled in terms of behaviours using openEHR archetypes. These form part of the openEHR methodology to develop unique applications [15]. The use of openEHR archetypes is gathering momentum for the development of next generation systems and the best

Table 9.2 An example of data and its contextual relationship

Data element (context)	Data
Age at admission	4
Eye colour	Brown
Diagnosis	Pneumonia or its ICD code
Site of wound	Left leg

possible use of clinical data. AI use of clinical data requires access to a large number of data points which can be made available through the use of these openly available openEHR methodologies [16], or possibly by large proprietary vendors making the best possible use of the latest cloud and AI capabilities. Either way it is critical that everyone adopts the same data standards. Nursing data needs to have well defined data models incorporating data elements that have defined meaning and format [17]. Such adoptions require national (ideally global) governance strategies.

The nursing profession does need to be aware that the level or degree of interoperability, is dependent upon the use of any combination of these information interchange schema and computing foundations in terms of how these are managing data exchange. Information interchange schema and computing foundations determins the degree or extent of interoperability achieved which has a flow on impact on the trustworthiness of the data used by AI technologies.

Trustworthiness is critical when AI is used for processing clinical data, or where results are used for point of care applications. It is important to remember that health professionals continue to be responsible for actions taken, irrespective of advice received from any AI system. Effective governance of clinical applications or the use of endorsement by an authoritative organization, such as the US Food and Drug Administration (FDA) or the Therapeutic Goods Administration (TGA) in Australia, improves trustworthiness. Greater tolerance regarding degree of accuracy is acceptable when data are only used by AI technologies for administrative purposes.

Figure 9.1 is a summary of some of these foundational concepts, shown as ranging from minimal ability of expressivity, as used for natural language processing, to the highest level of expressivity and therefore trustworthiness in terms of degree of accuracy and data quality. The use of AI technologies is all about knowledge management (Fig. 9.2).

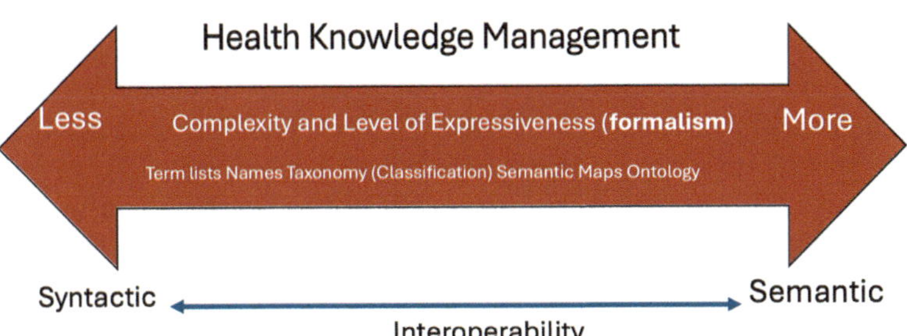

Fig. 9.2 Computable health knowledge management concepts and their relationships with AI technologies

AI Supporting Nursing Practice

An understanding of the many pre-requisites to be considered prior to the use of any AI technology is essential when considering how best to support any aspect of nursing practice. Nursing services are many and varied based on population demand, health services provided, clinical specialty and geographical location. Nursing documentation, workflows and the possible use of robotics vary accordingly.

Nursing Documentation and AI Support

Relevant, accurate, complete and timely information about a patient's care in any setting needs to be documented in every patient's health record. Nurses and midwives plan their care using the nursing process. The documentation of the nursing care plan using standard nursing terminologies (SNTs) is highly desirable as only then is it possible to make nursing's contribution visible statistically and provide the means to identify best practice from which evidence-based practice standards can be developed using data analytics.

> If you can't name it, you can't control it, finance it, research it, teach it, or put it into public policy [18]

Many countries require nursing documentation presented as care plans, although some large proprietary EMR systems only make checklists available to nurses for this purpose, which creates issues as the frequency and type of care-planning needs to differ between patients. Care plans need to be personalized based on each patient's health status and should not be a routine requirement for every shift. Another issue encountered is that few if any systems to date have access to sufficiently large nursing data sets to make AI use a reality. This is expected to change with a greater use of next generation systems which ideally separate data from the applications themselves.

Nursing activity recognition systems can automate documentation processes, including extracting key clinical information to generate personalised care plans, enabling caregivers to dedicate more time to patient-centred activities [19]. In its absence documentation time required has significantly increased in the US following the widespread introduction of EHRs [20]. It is critical for the nursing profession that unnecessary or meaningless documentation is eliminated. Regulatory and administrative data reporting needs to be automated and enabled by using data collected for clinical management purposes. Such measures are expected to reduce the documentation burden on nurses.

Next generation systems need to make use of a platform able to support robust, model-based abstraction of patient information (clinical models), recorded, stored and managed in a standardized manner. Their databases need to store electronically captured scalable data from multiple integrated EHRs compliant with the FAIR (findable, accessible, interoperable, reusable) principles [21]. This ensures semantic consistency across diverse healthcare systems and applications. A flexible and reusable framework can be provided by establishing a clear separation between clinical content and technical implementation able to access and retrieve data from a federated vendor/technology neutral data repository where data are compliant with standard nursing data models linked to standard terminologies. Only then is it possible to fully support nursing information needs and make use of AI technologies producing trustworthy outcomes.

Can or should AI be used to support nursing documentation? What are the potential benefits and risks? To answer these questions you need to evaluate your work environment to identify how this can best be achieved whilst ensuring patient safety and overall efficiency of AI use. Nursing informatics experts need to be part of the application design, implementation teams and manage potential risks.

Generative AI makes use of machine learning to create new content from images, video, audio or text. It is possible to generate personalized care-plans using generative AI making use of natural language processing with trustworthy data. One study [22] made use of a ChatGPT-based LLM tool, that was incorporated into their nursing information system in an ICU and a general ward to assist documentation. Nurses reported a significant reduction in time used to document plus improved workflow, accuracy, and a reduction in errors. Santos et al. [23] made use of a validated framework prompt to generate nursing care plan suggestions with ChatGPT, this demonstrated its potential value as a decision support tool for optimizing cancer care.

Many other similar AI technologies are available. Every tool is designed to best suit a specific purpose, some offer quality writing, others are more versatile, some are free, others require a subscription. Some organizations make these tools available for staff to use within their EHRs or organization portal.

Nursing Workflows in a Variety of Settings

Nursing workflow in any setting is the result of multiple factors, including technologies in use, communication processes, staff skill mix, location and availability of supplies, equipment, utility room locations relative to patients' point of care and nursing service delivery models adopted. AI tools designed to streamline nursing workflow need to be able to address the most time-consuming or troublesome influencing factor. Technologies in use include the availability of automated sphygmomanometers, thermometers, and other devices. One common technology in use is the electronic health record (EHR). The EHR user interfaces, ease of use and available functionalities determine if this application represents a nursing workflow bottleneck or supports workflow streamlining.

To make good use of AI technologies requires a thorough understanding of the key bottlenecks [24], only then is one able to choose the most appropriate AI technology able to address issues such as nurse staffing, the working environment, and/or the availability of devices in working order. The optimization or nursing workflows need to consider all of the above relative to nursing service demands which are dependent on the types and mix of health services provided and individual patients' severity of disease or injury. AI can be useful for nursing workload management [25], nursing resource allocation, supporting decision making, streamlining nursing processes, and can assist with communication between peers or departments. One does need to consider if alternatives may be more cost effective [26] prior to AI adoption.

One scoping review [27] found that the use of AI technologies such as machine learning and natural language processing provided better patient monitoring, better clinical decision making, more efficient use of resources and individualized treatment programs. AI may be able to improve workflow efficiency, reduce human error, automate some data entry, and enable nurses to spend more time interacting directly with patients.

Nursing Use of Robotics

Nurses tend to be in favour of adopting robotic technologies [28]. Robotic systems, like the Multi-purpose Intelligent Nurse Aid (MINA), assist in tasks such as patient mobility, walking support, and teleoperation, significantly reducing the physical burden on nurses and improving patient care. During the COVID-19 pandemic, robots played a vital role in reducing human exposure to infection by enabling remote operations [29]. Based on a patent study, robots for nursing care appear to be proliferating [30]. An ethnographic study [31] found that nursing care robots' design was largely influenced by popular scifi/cartoon contex rather than the result of thoughtful discussion about how best to embrace these technologies by the nursing profession.

In aged care, humanoid robots are providing social and emotional support to patients, alleviating loneliness and improving quality of life [32]. Socially Assistive Robots (SARs) show promise in nursing [33]. Surveys of nursing home administrators reveal a growing interest in using robots to augment caregiving, although concerns about cost, human interaction, and efficacy remain significant [34]. Compassionate care provided by humanoid robots requires nursing leadership with an ability to translate nursing, communication, computer science and engineering concepts into robotic care representations [35]. This requires collaborative efforts and ethical discourse considerations. Introducing robots into any care environment has a likely impact on the nursing role as such humanoid robots become part of the nursing care team. Nursing students need to be prepared accordingly to address a potential fear of being replaced by robots [36]. A systematic review [37] found that most robotic systems were in the development or testing phases. Nurses need to be educated to work with robotic designers and engineers enabling them to create user-friendly effective technologies that improve both patient care and nursing job satisfaction [28, 38].

Robotics can be cost-effective in the long run. While initial investments may be high, the automation of tasks and reduction in manual labor lead to significant cost savings over time. One needs to consider acquisition, installation, integration, safety management, staff training, support and maintenance including potential repair costs. Many robots require specialized programming to enable them to perform specific tasks. Potential returns include increased productivity and efficiency, reduced labour costs, improved quality control and enhanced safety. Efficiency for nurses means their ability to spend more time with patients resulting in outcome improvements.

Prior to AI tool development or acquisition it is useful to explore the workplace ecosystem to evaluate the readiness for AI implementation by determining current patient care and/or organizational performance risks and outcomes [26, 39] as well as staff readiness. This requires a careful analysis of all relevant factors and their relationships. The integration of robots may lead to a perceived or real loss of human touch, which is critical in nursing and midwifery where empathy and emotional support are paramount. Technical limitations also pose significant risks. Furthermore, the use of data-driven systems raises ethical and privacy concerns. Such systems must be compliant with legislative and regulatory requirements. Resistance to adoption is another challenge. There is a particular interest in making use of robots to support care for the elderly [40]. The future of robotics in nursing and midwifery is promising, with advancements in artificial intelligence and machine learning expected to drive innovation.

Robotics in nursing and midwifery represents a transformative advancement in healthcare. By improving efficiency, enhancing patient safety, and addressing workforce challenges, robotics offers immense potential to revolutionise care delivery. However, realising this potential requires careful planning, stakeholder engagement, and strategies to mitigate risks. As technology continues to evolve, the integration of robotics will play a pivotal role in shaping the future of nursing and midwifery.

Nurses, midwives and patients may hesitate to embrace robotics due to concerns about job displacement, loss of human interaction, and skepticism regarding the efficacy of these systems. Hybrid care models, where robots handle routine tasks while humans manage emotionally complex interactions, can help balance efficiency with empathy.

To maximise the benefits of robotics or any AI technology while mitigating risks, healthcare providers must adopt strategic implementation strategies. Engaging stakeholders, including nurses, midwives, and patients, during the design and deployment of robotic systems or AI technologies is crucial. This collaborative approach ensures that the technology addresses real-world needs and concerns, increasing acceptance and effectiveness. Phased deployment is another effective strategy. By starting with pilot programs, healthcare facilities can evaluate performance, gather feedback, and make necessary adjustments before scaling up. This approach minimises risks and ensures smoother integration of robotic systems or any other AI technology into existing workflows.

Patient Care and Ethical Considerations

> The primary rule for good policy, law and ethics is a sound understanding of the scientific data. [41]

Ethical practice is the result of an individual's own value system that influences their ability to know what is the right thing to do vs. what they have the right to do based on their interpretation of relevant policies, legislation and regulatory practices. Nurses are frequently confronted with having to make such decisions in the interest of their patient. Privacy legislation in fact may be the reason for doing harm. Ethics is a topic that every health and IT professional needs to have studied, although individual values about numerous ethical topics will vary making it difficult to gain consensus. Nurses need to engage with the emergence of 'roboethics', a new discourse for addressing AI robot technology [42] as the introduction of robotics to support any area of nursing practice introduces ontological and ethical issues that need to be fully explored.

The World Health Organization (WHO) has produced a publication of ethical principles for AI in Healthcare [43]. These are listed as:

1. Protect human autonomy
2. Promote human well-being and safety and the public interest
3. Ensure transparency, explainability and intelligibility
4. Foster responsibility and accountability
5. Ensure inclusiveness and equity
6. Promote AI that is responsive and sustainable

The Australian Medical Association (AMA) and the Australian College of Nursing (ACN) have each developed a position statement for AI [44, 45]. Another key aspect to be considered regarding all data use is patient privacy. Nurses need to recognize the delicate balance between the transformative potential of AI to improve patient care and the critical imperatives of data privacy, ethics, managing data bias and equitable healthcare access. Privacy challenges are associated with data robustness, legibility, scalability, adaptability, confidentiality, integrity, security and privacy versus utility. It is imperative that privacy and security legislation plus regulatory requirements reflect this balance between the public good and individual privacy.

There needs to be a distinction between identifiable data and de-identified data management practices. AI tools need to be compliant with the ISO/IEC 27559:2022 standard [46] which provides a framework for data de-identification that helps organizations mitigate risks associated with re-identification and the lifecycle of de-identified data. This standard suits any type of organization.

Separating the governance of demographic data and health data goes a long way towards the ability to achieve effective ethical data use. Demographic data governance is about identity management which should be a central function used for multiple purposes, such as residency, passports, driver licensing, eligibility for health or social service support, bank accounts and tax liabilities.

Another requirement is transparency regarding who is permitted to access and make use of which data for what purposes. Governance separation between identifiable and de-identified data does allow for re-identification when this is desired as a means to improve an individual's health status based on research findings, it is a useful protection against criminal or unethical use.

It is important for the nursing profession to be well represented in every entity, group, or committee with a mandate to manage AI in the healthcare system.

Outlook and Conclusions

The use of AI to support nursing practice is in its infancy. There is a strong need for nurses and midwives to build communities with an interest to drive AI research globally, to benefit not only the profession but those we care for as well. This will require sharing resources and multidisciplinary collaboration to not only support AI research but also to support professional development of the existing workforce and the education of new graduates.

This chapter presented a hierarchy of foundational AI functionalities that AI technologies make use of. When any area of nursing practice is identified as being repetitive or time consuming, one should consider which combination of AI functionalities is best suited to provide the desired beneficial support. For example, for AI to support care planning, the technology needs to be able to identify patterns, access and use historical data to predict likely outcomes and make recommendations. Such knowledge then forms the basis from which to determine AI potential.

It is critical for nurses and midwives to adopt a questioning approach and develop the ability to decompose their tasks and workflows as a precursor to exploring AI potential. An operational research capability enables nurses and midwives to contribute effectively to multidisciplinary collaborative AI developments as well to evaluation research once adopted to support nursing practice. All users of AI technologies need to be educationally prepared.

Useful Resources

Data First AI later presentation by Rachel Dunscombe UK. https://www.youtube.com/watch?v=ucDBjUgeK08

openEHR—100 videos and channels. https://www.youtube.com/hashtag/openehr

Nurse.org—AI in Nursing beyond the buzzwords to real world impact. https://www.youtube.com/watch?v=cT1fYYtjs4w

Review Questions

1. What is meant by 'functional capabilities' of AI technologies?
2. What are the fundamental pre-requisites for trustworthy beneficial AI use?
3. What information do you need to decide if it is beneficial to adopt AI to support nursing documentation?

4. How would you assess the ‘value’ of making use of a robot to support nursing practice?
5. What are the key ethical principles associated with AI use?
6. Which key factors need to be considered to mitigate risk?
7. Which factors would you consider as justifying the need for AI support?

Answers to Review Questions

1. The AI technology’s ability to perform specified tasks in order to achieve the desired outcome.
2. Beneficial AI use must comply with all applicable rules and regulations, including respect for privacy, adhere to agreed ethical principles and values, able to access a large amount of well governed quality data, e.g. unbiased and representative of the relevant knowledge domain, have technical robustness and safety.
3. Well defined issues associated with current documentation practices, such as errors, omissions, time required to document content, including content not required at point of care, with known quantifiable negative impacts. Such issues may be used as a business case to demonstrate the potential for a positive return on AI investments.
4. Robots can be of value if they can be shown to take on routine tasks enabling nursing to spend more time with their patients, and/or improve the quality of service delivery, improve patient independence and care outcomes.
5. Ethical principles associated with AI use include, transparency, fairness, accountability, privacy protection, non-discrimination, reliability, safety, human oversight, explainability, beneficial, contestability.
6. Risks can be effectively mitigated by ensuring that nurses and midwives receive proper education on the capabilities and limitations of AI. This includes ensuring AI complies with established ethical principles and user guidelines. Human judgement needs to be prioritized in critical situation. Users need to ensure that AI technologies were developed with diverse, representative and high quality data sets. Additionally, it is important that these technologies are able to access and make use of all relevant data to generate accurate responses prior to use.
7. AI support may be justified once potential benefits can be demonstrated such as:

    - clinical decisions enhanced to improve outcomes of care,
    - documentation requires less nursing time and is improved,
    - workflows are more efficient,
    - seamless access to complete data/information is more timely,
    - peer to peer communication is enhanced,
    - remote patient health status monitoring is improved,
    - administrative tasks are automated,
    - best practice guidelines are constantly updated and integrated with decision support systems,
    - virtual consultations are supported.

References

1. ISO-18104. Health informatics—categorial structures for representation of nursing practice in terminological systems. International Organisation of Standards. 2023. Available from: https://www.iso.org/standard/81132.html.
2. Hovenga E. Integrating a categorial structure for clinical practice into EHRs. Stud Health Technol Inform. 2024;310:74–8. https://doi.org/10.3233/SHTI230930.
3. ISO-13606-2. Health informatics – electronic health record communication – part 2: archetype interchange specification. International Organsiation for Standardisation. 2019 [cited 25 May 2019]. Available from: https://www.iso.org/standard/50119.html.
4. Peter S, Remer K. Wondering what AI actually is? Here are the 7 things it can do for you. The Conversation. 2024. Available from: https://theconversation.com/wondering-what-ai-actually-is-here-are-the-7-things-it-can-do-for-you-239843?utm_medium=email&utm_campaign=Latest%20from%20The%20Conversation%20for%20October%203%202024%20-%203115631793&utm_content=Latest%20from%20The%20Conversation%20for%20October%203%202024%20-%203115631793+CID_0025de6de78aa4b4d9ab254b142440ea&utm_source=campaign_monitor&utm_term=Wondering%20what%20AI%20actually%20is%20Here%20are%20the%207%20things%20it%20can%20do%20for%20you.
5. ISO-8373. Robotics – vocabulary. International Organsiation of Standards. 2021. Available from: https://www.iso.org/standard/75539.html.
6. O'Connor S, Yan Y, Thilo FJS, Felzmann H, Dowding D, Lee JJ. Artificial intelligence in nursing and midwifery: a systematic review. J Clin Nurs. 2023;32:2951–68. https://doi.org/10.1111/jocn.16478. Epub 2022 Jul 31.
7. openEHR. The future of digital health is open. openEHR International. Available from: https://www.openehr.org/.
8. CKM. openEHR clinical knowledge manager [cited 26 Sept 2018]. Available from: https://www.openehr.org/ckm/.
9. HL7-International. Fast healthcare interoperability resources specification (FHIR). Available from: https://www.hl7.org/fhir/overview.html.
10. Holmgren AJ, Esdar M, Hüsers J, Coutinho-Almeida J. Health information exchange: understanding the policy landscape and future of data interoperability. Yearb Med Inform. 2023;32:184–94. https://doi.org/10.1055/s-0043-1768719.
11. Hovenga EJS, Atalag K. Optimizing electronic health records to support artificial intelligence. AIH. 2024;1(3):10–25. https://doi.org/10.36922/aih.3056.
12. ISO/IEC-11179. Information technology – metadata registries (MDR) part1 framework. ISO. 2023. Available from: https://www.iso.org/obp/ui/#iso:std:iso-iec:11179:-1:en.
13. Hovenga Am EJS, Grain H. Trust in digital health- power of data myths. In: Almond H, Mather C, editors. Digital health-a transformative approach. Chatswood: Elsevier; 2024. p. 300.
14. OHDSI. Observational Health Data Sciences and Informatics [cited 11 Feb 2019]. Available from: https://www.ohdsi.org/.
15. Cardoso de Moraes JL, de Souza WL, Pires LF, do Prado AF. A methodology based on openEHR archetypes and software agents for developing e-health applications reusing legacy systems. Comput Methods Programs Biomed. 2016;134:267–87. https://doi.org/10.1016/j.cmpb.2016.07.013. Epub 2016 Jul 6.
16. Leslie H. openEHR archetype use and reuse within multilingual clinical data sets: case study. J Med Internet Res. 2020;22:e23361. https://doi.org/10.2196/23361.
17. Dugas M, Blumenstock M, Dittrich T, Eisenmann U, Feder SC, Fritz-Kebede F, Kessler LJ, Klass M, Knaup P, Lehmann CU, Merzweiler A, Niklas C, Pausch TM, Zental N, Ganzinger M. Next-generation study databases require FAIR, EHR-integrated, and scalable Electronic Data Capture for medical documentation and decision support. NPJ Digit Med. 2024;7:10. https://doi.org/10.1038/s41746-023-00994-6.
18. Clark J, Lang N. Nursing's next advance: an international classification for nursing practice. Int Nurs Rev. 1992;39:109–11, 128

19. Yadav S. Embracing artificial intelligence: revolutionizing nursing documentation for a better future. Cureus. 2024;16:e57725. https://doi.org/10.7759/cureus.57725.
20. Baumann LA, Baker J, Elshaug AG. The impact of electronic health record systems on clinical documentation times: a systematic review. Health Policy. 2018;122:827–36. https://doi.org/10.1016/j.healthpol.2018.05.014. Epub 2018 Jun 5.
21. GO-FAIR. FAIR principles. Available from: https://www.go-fair.org/fair-principles/.
22. Chen CJ, Liao CT, Tung YC, Liu CF. Enhancing healthcare efficiency: integrating ChatGPT in nursing documentation. Stud Health Technol Inform. 2024;316:851–2. https://doi.org/10.3233/SHTI240545.
23. Dos Santos FC, Johnson LG, Madandola OO, Priola KJB, Yao Y, Macieira TGR, Keenan GM. An example of leveraging AI for documentation: ChatGPT-generated nursing care plan for an older adult with lung cancer. J Am Med Inform Assoc. 2024;31:2089–96. https://doi.org/10.1093/jamia/ocae116.
24. Al Moteri M, Aljuaid J, Alsufyani B, Alghamdi A, Althobiti ES, Althagafi A. Bottleneck factors impacting nurses' workflow and the opportunity to prioritize improvement efforts: factor analysis. BMC Nurs. 2024;23:640. https://doi.org/10.1186/s12912-024-02311-2.
25. Hovenga E, Lowe C. Measuring capacity to care using nursing data. London: Elsevier, Academic Press; 2020.
26. Hovenga E, Hazelton LM, Britnell S. Using six sigma lean and other tools for measuring quality. In: Saba V, McCormick K, editors. Essentials of nursing informatics. New York: McGraw-Hill; 2019. In press.
27. Alanazi MS, Al-Otaibi MB, Alzurayq JI, Alessa LM, Alotaibi ASD, MuqbilAlthobaiti MA, Zaki H, Alsayafi A, Alaqil AS, Alasmari AAM. Effectiveness of artificial intelligence in resource management and nursing workflow: a scoping review. J Int Crisis Risk Commun Res. 2024;7:99–111.
28. Georgadarellis GL, Cobb T, Vital CJ, Sup FC 4th. Nursing perceptions of robotic technology in healthcare: a pretest-posttest survey analysis using an educational video. IISE Trans Occup Ergon Hum Factors. 2024;12:68–83. https://doi.org/10.1080/24725838.2024.2323061.
29. Kodur KC, Rajpathak K, Rajavenkatanarayanan A, Kyrarini M, Makedon F. Towards a multi-purpose robotic nursing assistant. Cornell University; 2021. https://doi.org/10.48550/arXiv.2106.03683.
30. Frazier RM, Carter-Templeton H, Wyatt TH, Wu L. Current trends in robotics in nursing patents-a glimpse into emerging innovations. Comput Inform Nurs. 2019;37:290–7. https://doi.org/10.1097/CIN.0000000000000538.
31. Eriksson H, Salzmann-Erikson M. The digital generation and nursing robotics: a netnographic study about nursing care robots posted on social media. Nurs Inq. 2017;24:e12165. https://doi.org/10.1111/nin.12165.
32. Tobis S, Piasek-Skupna J, Neumann-Podczaska A, Suwalska A, Wieczorowska-Tobis K. The effects of stakeholder perceptions on the use of humanoid robots in care for older adults: postinteraction cross-sectional study. J Med Internet Res. 2023;25:e46617. https://doi.org/10.2196/46617.
33. Mistry M. Exploring robotic nursing: a comprehensive systematic review of socially assistive robots within the healthcare professions. J Community Health Nurs. 2025;42(3):155–68. https://doi.org/10.1080/07370016.2024.2436886.
34. Imtiaz R, Khan A. Perceptions of humanoid robots in caregiving: a study of skilled nursing home and long term care administrators. Cornell University; 2024. https://doi.org/10.48550/arXiv.2401.02105.
35. Hernandez JP. Compassionate care with autonomous AI humanoid robots in future healthcare delivery: a multisensory simulation of next-generation models. Biomimetics. 2024;9(11):687. https://doi.org/10.3390/biomimetics9110687.
36. Wong P, Brand G, Dix S, Choo D, Foley P, Lokmic-Tomkins Z. Pre-registration nursing students' perceptions of digital health technology on the future of nursing: a qualitative exploratory study. Nurse Educ. 2024;49:E208–12. https://doi.org/10.1097/NNE.0000000000001591.

37. Ohneberg C, Stöbich N, Warmbein A, Rathgeber I, Mehler-Klamt AC, Fischer U, Eberl I. Assistive robotic systems in nursing care: a scoping review. BMC Nurs. 2023;22:72. https://doi.org/10.1186/s12912-023-01230-y.
38. Gonzalo de Diego B, González Aguña A, Fernández Batalla M, Herrero Jaén S, Sierra Ortega A, Barchino Plata R, Jiménez Rodríguez ML, Santamaría García JM. Competencies in the robotics of care for nursing robotics: a scoping review. Healthcare (Basel). 2024;12:617. https://doi.org/10.3390/healthcare12060617.
39. Hovenga E. Nursing work measurement methods and their use. In: Hovenga E, Lowe C, editors. Measuring capacity to care using nursing data. Cambridge, MA: Elsevier Inc.; 2019.
40. Sawik B, Tobis S, Baum E, Suwalska A, Kropińska S, Stachnik K, Pérez-Bernabeu E, Cildoz M, Agustin A, Wieczorowska-Tobis K. Robots for elderly care: review, multi-criteria optimization model and qualitative case study. Healthcare (Basel). 2023;11:1286. https://doi.org/10.3390/healthcare11091286.
41. Kirby HJM. Bioethics and democracy – a fundamental question. In: Charlesworth M, editor. Life, death, genes and ethics: biotechnology and bioethics. Crows Nest: ABC Books; 1989. p. 145.
42. Wangi K, Birriel B, Smith C. Perspectives: nursing roboethics: ethical issues for artificial intelligence robots, nurses' roles and the future. J Res Nurs. 2024;29:186–90. https://doi.org/10.1177/17449871241231385.
43. WHO. Ethics and governance of artificial intelligence for health: WHO guidance. Geneva: World health Organisation; 2021. Available from: https://www.who.int/publications/i/item/9789240029200
44. AMA. Position statement: artifical intelligence in healthcare. 2023. Available from: https://www.ama.com.au/sites/default/files/2023-08/Artificial%20Intelligence%20in%20Healthcare%20-%20AMA.pdf.
45. ACN. Artificial intelligence- position statement. Canberra: Australian College of Nursing; 2024. Available from: https://www.acn.edu.au/advocacy-policy/position-statement-artificial-intelligence.
46. ISO/IEC-27559. Information security, cybersecurity and privacy protection – privacy enhancing data de-identification framework. 2022. Available from: https://www.iso.org/standard/71677.html.

Part IV
Challenges and Background

Chapter 10
Navigating Data Diversity and Equity in Healthcare with AI

Giovanni Rubeis

Learning Objectives
- To understand the link between bias and health equity.
- To distinguish different types of bias.
- To understand the concept of health equity.
- To investigate ways of diversifying data.
- To explore strategies for reducing bias and safeguarding health equity.

Key Terms
- Artificial intelligence
- Bias
- Bioethics
- Health equity
- Machine learning
- Thick data

Summary
This paper addresses health equity as a major factor for bridging the gap between medical AI and clinical practice. Addressing and mitigating bias is key for reducing existing health disparities and preventing their exacerbation through AI-technologies. I argue that the gap between artificial and human intelligence is one potential cause of exacerbating health disparities through bias. In turn, bias causes a gap between the possibilities of AI in healthcare and its clinical application. Reconciling human and artificial intelligence through technical bias mitigation, human-centered AI and thick data approaches, and regulations, is necessary to enable equity in an AI-based healthcare setting.

G. Rubeis (✉)
Institute of Ethics and History of Medicine, University of Greifswald, Greifswald, Germany
e-mail: giovanni.rubeis@med.uni-greifswald.de

U. H. Hübner et al. (eds.), *Bridging Artificial and Human Intelligence*, Health Informatics, https://doi.org/10.1007/978-3-032-11938-4_10

Introduction

The big data approach is the new paradigm in healthcare. For decades, evidence-based medicine (EBM) has been the standard approach, meaning that clinical decisions ought to be based on the best available scientific evidence. This implies a hierarchy of medical knowledge in terms of evidence, starting with personal experience and intuition at the very bottom to scientific knowledge provided by randomized clinical trials (RCTs) and meta-reviews as the highest form of evidence. The big data approach changes this paradigm in that it focuses more on individual health data. An RCT for example represents data from hundreds, sometimes thousands of patients or test subjects and analyses it in a statistical manner, e.g. to determine the outcomes of a procedure or the ideal dosage of a drug. This average patient is a statistical fiction and differs from the individual patient a doctor is faced with. It is one of the core medical tasks to bridge the epistemic gap between scientific knowledge and the individual patient, their concrete needs, resources, and characteristics. The advantage of the big data approach is its focus on the individual instead of large cohorts. The aim is to gain as much individual health data as possible, ideally combining physiological with behavioral and environmental data. Processing, combining, and analyzing this multimodal data enables more accurate models of an individual's health situation and thus provides a better evidence-basis for clinical decision-making. This includes not only the representation of a person's health, but also enabling predicative analysis in order to predict future events, e.g. the onset of disease, and thus implementing preventive measures early on.

The big data approach only works when sufficient high-quality data is available. It is trivial to note that data models are only as good as the data they are based on, but it is nevertheless an essential factor in healthcare. Data has to be accurate so as to minimize error margins, which may have serious consequences. In the same way, the machine learning techniques applied to the data have to be fitting and sound. Otherwise, even high-quality data cannot be transformed into a valid model.

The crucial risk in this context is bias. This term is used in different contexts or disciplines and has different meanings. In informatics and data science, bias simply refers to a variety of possible measurement errors that cause a faulty representation in data models [1]. In this view, bias is a statistical issue that occurs when the number of variables is too limited to give an adequate representation of a phenomenon or the data set itself is simply inadequate. But bias also plays a key role in ethical considerations of the big data approach in healthcare. In fact, the bias problem has been considered as the crucial ethical issue regarding the use of machine learning applications in healthcare [2]. In a broader understanding, bias is the inadequate reduction of complexity regarding the characteristics of individuals or social groups. It is a stereotypical and mostly discriminatory view that either defines a person or group by a certain trait or ignores certain characteristic traits that are indispensable to fully understand their situation. In healthcare, the main risk of bias is that it undermines health equity, the principle to treat each individual according to their specific needs and resources. Bias often leads to outcomes that deprive individuals or social groups of the treatment they need, thus exacerbating social discrimination. One could therefore say that the basic problem we are facing here is that bias as the failure to acknowledge or account for diversity undermines health equity and thus also the quality of care.

In the following, I will discuss this problem as well as possible solutions. In a first step, I will explain the concept of equity in the healthcare context. In a second step, I will outline different types of bias and their causes. In a final step, I will discuss several strategies for dealing with the bias problem, followed by a conclusion. In my view, addressing the bias problem as a threat to health equity is an essential necessity for bridging the gap between healthcare AI as a concept and its application in clinical practice.

Health Equity

The concept of equity differs from its close relative equality, although both are sometimes confused. Equality implies considering or treating individuals as equal. For example, all individuals are equal in regard to basic human rights. Treating people equally is thus a major aspect of justice. However, in some cases, simply treating everyone in the same way is not enough. Equity accounts for the fact that sometimes the differences between individuals, their specific characteristics, needs, and resources have to be considered in order to make just decisions. Aristotle found an early definition for this specific type of justice, which requires treating equals equally and unequals unequally [3]. In healthcare, equity is essential, since medical treatment and care requires considering individual factors. Not all people have the same health needs or resources to deal with health issues. Hence, they have to be treated according to their specific characteristics.

Another important terminological distinction is that between health differences and health disparities [4]. Whereas health differences between individuals are a result of the natural, i.e. genetic or physiological, variety of human beings, health disparities are man-made. They result from systemic or structural inequalities, which means processes, rules, and practices within a healthcare system that do not account for individual health needs, either intentionally or unintentionally. Health disparities may imply denying people access to healthcare or withhold resources from them due to their age, gender, ethnicity, sexual identity, religion, disability, or socio-economic status. These social determinants of health, i.e. non-medical factors that shape an individual's health as well as their access to healthcare, have to be considered when thinking about equity and justice [5]. It is important to note that health disparities are not only relevant in the context of medicine and healthcare. Since health can be seen as a transcendental good, a necessary condition for fulfilling one's life plan, health disparities may affect the opportunities of an individual to participate in society and live a fulfilling life [4, 6]. Hence health disparities are also a matter of social justice [7].

Whereas equality implies granting the same (chances, services, resources) to all, equity acknowledges the fact that individuals start from different positions. Social determinants like age, gender, ethnicity, or socio-economic status shape the health needs and resources of individuals. Structural factors like racism or discrimination also play an important role in this respect. These determinants and factors also affect access to health services as well as health outcomes, creating health disparities that are defined as avoidable differences between individuals or groups. The principle of equity implies to compensate these avoidable differences by ensuring that needs are catered to according to the specific social situation of an individual. A major factor that undermines health equity and produces or exacerbates health disparities is bias.

Bias

Bias has been identified as a risk in computer-based data analysis as early as the 1990s. Friedman and Nissenbaum [8] distinguish between preexisting bias, referring to social practices, attitudes, and institutions, technical bias, which results from operational mechanisms of computer systems, and emergent bias. i.e. the outcomes of computer-based data analysis. That means that bias may be in the data or may be caused by algorithms and machine learning or be the result of data use. Accordingly, one can identify three levels of bias, *data bias, algorithmic bias,* and *outcome bias* [9]. *Data bias* means that the data to be analyzed or the training data with which algorithms are trained are biased. For example, if a computer vision software for detecting melanoma, a now common application in dermatology, has been trained exclusively with pictures of white skin it will most certainly fail to correctly identify melanoma on darker skin tones. *Algorithmic bias* occurs when the algorithms are built on parameters that exclude certain individuals or groups. Many machine learning techniques require defining target variables and class labels, or, in other words, what to look for and how to sort the results into distinct groups [10]. If target variables and class labels are designed in a way so that they ignore certain traits or overemphasize others, those individuals or groups who have or lack certain traits will not be detected by the algorithm. This is also called the signal problem, since signals from certain individuals or groups are not detected and hence, they are not represented in algorithmic models [11]. *Outcome bias* is a consequence of one or both other types of bias. When clinical decision-making is based on biased data models, either due to data bias or algorithmic bias, the outcome, e.g. choosing a therapeutic option, will also be biased.

In most cases, these three levels are not isolated from each other; rather, we are dealing with a bias cascade [9]. There is a striking example for the bias cascade discussed in the study by Obermeyer and colleagues [12]. The authors investigated an algorithm in the US-healthcare system tasked with sorting patients into risk groups. Depending on their risk level, patients were granted access to healthcare services. The main parameter the algorithm was built on was health costs. The algorithm worked on the basic correlation between health costs invested into a patient in the past and the risk for needing healthcare services later on. The algorithm had learned that the more costs have been invested into a patient, the more likely they will be to require further health costs in the future, which means that they are sorted into a higher risk group and thus have easier access to healthcare services. The algorithm was "unaware", to use an anthropomorphic term solely for the purpose of clarification, of the fact that less health costs are invested into African-Americans for socio-political reasons. Hence it did not account for the structural discrimination of this group within the US-healthcare system. The result was that the majority of African-Americans were assigned a lesser risk label and thus services were withheld from them although they had a clear health need. This exemplifies the workings of the bias cascade. It starts with biased data that does not account for the structural discrimination of a certain social group but presents this simply as a fact. This biased data is then used for training an algorithm that focuses on biased parameters, in this example health costs. Finally, by incorrectly assigning risk labels, the decision-making based on this algorithm leads to a continuation or even exacerbation of existing health disparities.

The bias problem related to AI in healthcare has severe ethical consequences, especially regarding equity [2]. Bias on different levels or in the form of a cascade undermines health equity because it distorts the representation of certain individuals or groups in data models. This has been referred to as epistemic injustice [13] or ontic occlusion [11]. Ontic occlusion describes the connection between epistemic practices and normative outcomes. To put it simply, a data model that ignores a certain trait, either due to data bias or algorithmic bias, will not represent those individuals with that trait. If these individuals are not represented by the model, they become virtually invisible. Their exclusion from the data results in a social exclusion, since they are not part of social practices, in our case healthcare services. This epistemic injustice leads to social injustice, since the health needs of these individuals are ignored, thus exacerbating existing health disparities. Chan and colleagues speak of an "equity gap" in AI-based healthcare [14]. Bridging this gap is essential to use AI for the benefit of patients.

A comparison might be in place here. In order for drugs to be deployed, their effectiveness and risks for the population they are aimed for have to be tested. Pharmacovigilance, as it is often called, requires evaluating and validating drugs in terms of outcomes and safety. In the same way, *algorithmovigilance* could be understood as a combination of strategies for evaluating, monitoring, and preventing negative outcomes of AI-based treatments [15]. An important aspect here is that technical means alone are insufficient to achieve this. As we have seen, bias does not only result from technical issues like choosing the wrong statistical method or applying such a method incorrectly. There are also systemic factors that may cause bias. For one, bias might be already in the data, e.g. the data set for training algorithms. Furthermore, bias may occur from the interaction between humans and algorithms, for example the selection of variables and other parameters as in the example of the biased algorithm in the US-healthcare system above. Therefore, it is imperative to include social practices and structural factors as targets for debiasing strategies.

Strategies

Given the fact that bias may occur in various forms, i.e. as data bias, algorithmic bias, and outcome bias, strategies for overcoming it must be equally versatile. One could distinguish between technical and non-technical approaches according to their means as well as targets. Bridging the equity gap requires both types of strategies.

Technical Approaches

Technical approaches aim to eliminate or mitigate bias by improving statistical techniques for data analysis. The label algorithmic fairness is often used to describe various strategies for bias mitigation in machine learning [2]. These strategies can be applied in the *pre-processing, in-processing,* and *post-processing phase* of data analysis [16].

In *pre-processing,* data bias is the main target. As we have seen, one of the main factors here is selection bias and the signal problem that results from it. When a social group is underrepresented in the training data for an algorithm, the resulting data model will not contain relevant information about said group. Thus, signals that highlight the situation of this group will be muted and an ontic occlusion might occur, resulting in a perpetuation or even exacerbation of existing health disparities. The sample can be addressed through technical means, i.e. statistical approaches. One example is importance weighting, whereby data from underrepresented groups is assigned a stronger weight, i.e. significance in the analysis [16]. Sampling methods can also be applied, which entails adding or removing samples to the initial sample or reconsidering their significance [17]. Resampling refers to correcting the original data by obtaining more diverse subsamples that account for minority groups. Relabeling means to change the ground truth labels [16]. In perturbation, the aim is to adjust the values so that their distributions are closer together, whereby the ranking remains the same. This could be done in an iterative way by identifying the attribute most likely to be biased and then transforming it until the bias of the model is below a defined threshold [17].

In-processing bias mitigation focuses on confounding errors that occur when protected attributes are used as shortcuts for model prediction [16]. One way is to change the learning algorithm's loss function, a statistical function that indicates how well an algorithm performs by mapping the error margin between estimated values and true values of a data model [17]. The lower the loss function, the more precise the algorithm. By adding a regulation term, discriminations of the loss function, i.e. higher error margins, are penalized. In addition to this so-called regulation, constraints can be applied, which means defining a specific bias level as a limit during training. Another approach is adversarial learning, whereby classification models are trained to predict ground truth values while the adversary model exploits fairness issues. In adjusted learning, external decision makers intervene and change the algorithmic procedure. The classification model becomes selective by learning to abstain from making predictions in specific cases. The downside of in-processing approaches is that they might reduce overall model performance [16].

Post-processing bias mitigation focuses on modifying the output of models that have already been trained [17]. This approach aims to revise outcomes and recalibrate algorithms in case of error [18]. This may entail input correction of the training data, classifier correction, or output correction, the latter of which implies modifying the predicted labels [17]. As with in-processing bias mitigation, also post-processing approaches may reduce the performance of an algorithm and thus the accuracy of the model [16].

This list is not complete and combined approaches are feasible. It nevertheless shows that there are various technical approaches in terms of modifying either the data or the statistical methods for mitigating bias. However, the complexity of the bias problem calls for additional approaches, since bias is not merely a technical issue. As we have seen, bias often results not primarily from misguided application of statistical techniques, but rather from systemic conditions and social practices. Hence, non-technical strategies for bias mitigation are also required.

Non-technical Approaches

Human-centered AI (HCAI) is an approach that aims to shift the focus from algorithms and machines to humans, their needs and values [19]. This focus shift means to not only evaluate AI by measuring algorithmic performance but also considering the impact of AI-technologies on users and society as a whole. User observation, stakeholder engagement, usability testing, and continuing evaluation of human performance in AI-use are crucial tools in this regard. The basic idea is to design AI-technologies so that they enable and augment human performance instead of substituting humans through fully automatized processes. A high level of automatization has to go hand-in-hand with high levels of human control, following HCAI. Applications have to be reliable safe and trustworthy, which can be achieved for the most part by stakeholder engagement and participation in the design and development pathway.

Turchi and colleagues [20] demonstrate what this means in the healthcare context by applying HCAI methods to an AI-as-a-service platform that enables broader access to customized diagnostic and rehabilitative processes. The challenge here is to create a technology that is adaptable, fosters trust, and is tailored to the personal needs of patients while at the same time fitting seamlessly with the clinical workflow. In other words, bridging the gap between artificial and human intelligence is key to design a system that enables a more democratized access to healthcare services. Turchi and colleagues [20] used stakeholder workshops, user journey maps, and post-workshop questionnaires to assess human-AI interaction in the light of ethical principles. The researchers chose endocrinology and child neuropsychiatry as use cases, involving healthcare professionals from different experience levels as participants. This exchange of perspectives provided collective insights into expected challenges such as technology deployment, dynamic data utilization, clinical collaboration, and bias mitigation. By balancing technological innovation with human-centric considerations, the researchers provided a method for designing an inclusive AI-technology based on combining human and artificial intelligence.

Thick data refers to an approach that acknowledges the social embeddedness of data genesis and data collection [2, 21]. Following this view, data does not speak for itself but needs to be contextualized with the social background within which it was generated as well as the social practices surrounding data collection. When data is isolated from this context, meaning and crucial information is lost, which may undermine the very goal of data-intensive medicine, i.e. personalization and better health outcomes. One important aspect in this regard is the needs and resources of specific social groups, which often help to understand why data is the way it is. Hence, ethnographic approaches like interviews, social media analysis, or stakeholder workshops could be used to contextualize health data and thus overcome the above-mentioned signal problem [2, 22]. That such a strategy is technically feasible has been shown already [22, 23].

Medical device regulation is essential in providing safety and protecting patients against harm. This is also an approach that applies to AI-technologies in healthcare, be it AI elements in a device or stand-alone software [24]. Analytic validity, clinical validity, and clinical utility of AI-technologies are the focus here. Usually, medical devices are evaluated by risk, meaning that the limits of use as well as the level of scrutiny in evaluating devices depends on the risk-level assigned to a device or software. Regulatory approaches especially target representativeness and require disclosures in regard to data quality. Furthermore, continuous monitoring of algorithm performance as well as developer liability are major aspects here [24].

The fast-paced emergence of AI-technology in healthcare has shown that medical device regulation is insufficient for covering all aspects of this new technology. Hence, broader regulatory approaches are required. Especially two regulatory acts are worth mentioning here. The EU AI Act (AIA) was adopted by all member states in 2024. AIA aims to foster human-centered and trustworthy AI, focusing on protecting the health, safety, and fundamental rights of individuals [25]. It classifies AI in three risk classes from low to high risk. The important aspect here is that AIA goes beyond medical product regulation, since it also pertains to applications that are not specifically designed for medical purposes, such as ChatGPT. Its main focus is on averting rights-based harm towards individuals or groups, i.e. undermining their rights in society such as participating in the democratic process [26]. One could argue that this also pertains to equity in healthcare, since health inequities mitigate an individual's capability of social participation.

In the USA, the Department of Health and Human Services and the Office of the National Coordinator within Department of Health and Human Services have implemented regulations targeting AI-driven discrimination in healthcare [24]. These regulations focus on algorithmic transparency, especially regarding algorithmic performance, to enable responsible AI development and use [27]. This is an addition to existing regulations of medical devices under the Food Drug and Cosmetic Act (FDCA) by the Food and Drug Administration (FDA) [24].

The main focus of regulations in both jurisdictions is protecting the rights of individuals through transparency of algorithms, representativeness as well as diversity of data, and risk management [24, 26, 28]. This is especially important, since transparency regarding the development, testing, implementation, and evaluation of algorithms is a major principle within the debate on bridging the equity gap [29].

However, one crucial problem of regulatory strategies that aim to foster data diversity is the very concept itself. It is very difficult to define what diversity means in each use case or what extent of diversity is needed [24]. Another issue here is to balance these regulations with existing laws on data protection like the General Data Protection Regulation (GDPR) in the EU or the Health Insurance Portability and Accountability Act (HIPAA) in the USA that limit health data collection [24]. A particular difficulty arises when a genuinely horizontal legislation like AIA intersects with vertical regulations for specific sectors such as medical device regulation [28]. Conflicts or unnecessary duplication of legislation may be the results.

This shows that regulatory measures, although indispensable, are not to be seen as a silver bullet. Enabling health equity through bias mitigation and data diversity needs a combination of different approaches and strategies.

Outlook and Conclusions

This paper addresses health equity as a crucial factor for bridging the gap between AI-based healthcare technologies and clinical practice. Addressing and mitigating bias is key for reducing existing health disparities and preventing their exacerbation through AI-technologies. When looking closer at these issues as well as the strategies for overcoming them, it becomes clear that bridging the gap between artificial and human intelligence plays a crucial role in this regard. Bias mitigating requires human interference in algorithmic processes, e.g. by validating parameters such as variables and group classifiers as well as scrutinizing statistical methods and machine learning techniques. Furthermore, diversifying data, especially training data for algorithms, is a crucial task that requires human engagement. Contextualizing data by considering causalities, e.g. between structural discrimination and poor health outcomes for specific social groups, is an important human contribution. Hence, one could say that the gap between artificial and human intelligence is a major factor for the risk of exacerbating health disparities through bias. In turn, bias is a crucial factor that causes the gap between the technical possibilities of AI in healthcare and its real-world application in clinical practice. Therefore, reconciling human artificial intelligence through bias mitigation, HCAI and thick data approaches, transparency and education, and regulation, is necessary to enable equity in an AI-based healthcare setting.

Useful Resources

ASP belong, an EU-funded international research project based on a collaborative approach to ensure data diversity and include stakeholders in the development of a gamified augmented reality mental health intervention. https://www.augmentedsocialplay.com/

Resources and further information on health equity by the World Health Organization (WHO): https://www.who.int/health-topics/health-equity#tab=tab_1

Review Questions

1. What does health equity mean?
2. Which types of bias are there?
3. How does bias affect health equity?
4. What are possible strategies to overcome bias and to enable health equity?

Answers to Review Questions

1. Treating patients according to their specific health needs.
2. Data bias, algorithmic bias, outcome bias.
3. Bias distorts the representation of certain individuals or groups in data models which leads to epistemic injustice or ontic occlusion.
4. Technical bias mitigation, human-centered AI, thick data, and regulatory approaches.

References

1. Mitchell S, Potash E, Barocas S, D'amour A, Lum K. Algorithmic fairness: choices, assumptions, and definitions. Ann Rev Stat Appl. 2021;8:141–63. https://doi.org/10.1146/annurev-statistics-042720-125902.
2. Rubeis G. Ethics of medical AI. Cham: Springer Nature; 2024.
3. Aristotle N. Ethics, translated by Bartlett RC and Collins SD. Chicago: University of Chicago Press; 2011.
4. Braveman PA, Kumanyika S, Fielding J, Laveist T, Borrell LN, Manderscheid R, Troutman A. Health disparities and health equity: the issue is justice. Am J Public Health. 2011;101(Suppl 1):149–55. https://doi.org/10.2105/AJPH.2010.300062.
5. Daniels N. Just health: meeting health needs fairly. Cambridge: Cambridge University Press; 2007.
6. Sen A. Why health equity? Health Econ. 2002;11:659–66. https://doi.org/10.1002/hec.762.
7. Ruger JP. Health and social justice. Lancet. 2004;364:1075–80. https://doi.org/10.1016/S0140-6736(04)17064-5.
8. Friedman B, Nissenbaum H. Bias in computer systems. ACM Trans Inf Syst. 1996;14:330–47.
9. Alhasan A. Bias in medical artificial intelligence. Bull R Coll Surg Engl. 2021;103:302–5.
10. Barocas S, Selbst AD. Big data's disparate impact. Calif Law Rev. 2016;104:671–732.
11. Mittelstadt BD, Floridi L. The ethics of big data: current and foreseeable issues in biomedical contexts. Sci Eng Ethics. 2016;22:303–41. https://doi.org/10.1007/s11948-015-9652-2.
12. Obermeyer Z, Powers B, Vogeli C, Mullainathan S. Dissecting racial bias in an algorithm used to manage the health of populations. Science. 2019;366:447–53. https://doi.org/10.1126/science.aax2342.
13. Fricker M. Epistemic injustice: power and the ethics of knowing. Oxford: Oxford University Press; 2007.

14. Chan SCC, Neves AL, Majeed A, Faisal A. Bridging the equity gap towards inclusive artificial intelligence in healthcare diagnostics. Br Med J. 2024;384:q490. https://doi.org/10.1136/bmj.q490.
15. Embi PJ. Algorithmovigilance—advancing methods to analyze and monitor artificial intelligence–driven health care for effectiveness and equity. JAMA Netw Open. 2021;4(4):e214622. https://doi.org/10.1001/jamanetworkopen.2021.4622.
16. Chen RJ, Wang JJ, Williamson DFK, et al. Algorithmic fairness in artificial intelligence for medicine and healthcare. Nat Biomed Eng. 2023;7:719–42. https://doi.org/10.1038/s41551-023-01056-8.
17. Hort M, Chen Z, Zhang J, Sarro F, Harman M. Bias mitigation for machine learning classifiers: a comprehensive survey. ACM J Respons Comput. 2022;1:1–52. https://doi.org/10.1145/3631326.
18. Kordzadeh N, Ghasemaghaei M. Algorithmic bias: review, synthesis, and future research directions. Eur J Inf Syst. 2022;31:388–409. https://doi.org/10.1080/0960085X.2021.1927212.
19. Shneiderman B. Human-centered AI. Oxford: Oxford University Press; 2022.
20. Turchi T, Prencipe G, Malizia A, Filogna S, Latrofa F, Sgandurra G. Pathways to democratized healthcare: envisioning human-centered AI-as-a-service for customized diagnosis and rehabilitation. Artif Intell Med. 2024;151:102850. https://doi.org/10.1016/j.artmed.2024.102850.
21. Wang T. Big data needs thick data. Ethnography Matters Blog [online], May 2013. Available at: https://ethnographymatters.net/blog/2013/05/13/big-data-needs-thick-data/. Accessed 17 Nov 2025.
22. Fiaidhi J. Envisioning insight-driven learning based on thick data analytics with focus on healthcare. IEEE Access. 2020;8:114998–5004. https://doi.org/10.1109/ACCESS.2020.2995763.
23. Nguyen M, Eulalio T, Marafino BJ, Rose C, Chen JH, Baiocchi M. Thick data analytics (TDA): an iterative and inductive framework for algorithmic improvement. Am Stat. 2024;78(4):456–64. https://doi.org/10.1080/00031305.2024.2327535.
24. McKibbin KJ, Popejoy AB, Shabani M. Reconciling diversity in health and genomic data collection with the regulation of AI in clinical genomics. Genet Med. 2024;26(7):101127. https://doi.org/10.1016/j.gim.2024.101127.
25. European Parliament. Artificial Intelligence Act. 2024. https://www.europarl.europa.eu/doceo/document/TA-9-2024-0138_EN.pdf. Last access: 20 Dec 2024.
26. Cupać J, Sienknecht M. Regulate against the machine: how the EU mitigates AI harm to democracy. Democratization. 2024;31(5):1067–90. https://doi.org/10.1080/13510347.2024.2353706.
27. US Department of Health and Human Services (HHS). Health data, technology, and interoperability: certification program updates, algorithm transparency, and information sharing. Final rule. 2023. https://www.healthit.gov/sites/default/files/page/2023-12/hti-1-final-rule.pdf. Last access: 20 Dec 2024.
28. Busch F, Kather JN, Johner C, Moser M, Truhn D, Adams LC, Bressem KK. Navigating the European Union Artificial Intelligence Act for Healthcare. NPJ Digit Med. 2024;7:210. https://doi.org/10.1038/s41746-024-01213-6.
29. Murphy A, Bowen K, Naqa IME, Yoga B, Green BL. Bridging health disparities in the data-driven world of artificial intelligence: a narrative review. J Racial Ethn Health Disparities. 2024;12(4):2367–79. https://doi.org/10.1007/s40615-024-02057-2.

Chapter 11
Regulatory Frameworks for AI: The Legal and Ethical Perspective

Volker Lüdemann

Learning Objectives
- To understand the key ethical, legal, and regulatory challenges of AI in healthcare.
- To critically analyze and compare AI regulatory frameworks in the EU and the U.S., highlighting their similarities, differences, and implications for healthcare professionals, policymakers, and AI developers.
- To gain a comprehensive understanding of major legal frameworks, including the AI Act, MDR, GDPR, and FDA regulations.
- To identify and assess regulatory gaps related to AI governance, liability, and health data protection in healthcare.
- To evaluate the role of data protection laws (e.g., GDPR, HIPAA) and their impact on responsible AI-driven healthcare systems.
- To explore emerging trends in AI regulation and assess their potential impact on medical practice and healthcare innovation.

Key Terms
- Artificial intelligence (AI) in healthcare
- General Data Protection Regulation (GDPR)
- EU Artificial Intelligence (AI) Act
- Health Insurance Portability and Accountability Act (HIPAA)
- Medical Device Regulation (MDR)
- Ethical guidelines for trustworthy AI
- Liability for AI in healthcare
- Black box problem in AI
- Algorithmic bias in healthcare AI

V. Lüdemann (✉)
Osnabrück University of Applied Sciences, Osnabrück, Germany

U. H. Hübner et al. (eds.), *Bridging Artificial and Human Intelligence*, Health Informatics, https://doi.org/10.1007/978-3-032-11938-4_11

Summary
The regulation of artificial intelligence (AI) in healthcare must strike a balance between technological innovation and legal as well as ethical requirements. While the European Union (EU) employs a preventive and standardized approach through the AI Act, the Medical Device Regulation (MDR), and the General Data Protection Regulation (GDPR), the United States (US) adopts industry-specific and more flexible regulations. Key challenges include governing adaptive AI systems, ensuring the use of large health data sets while maintaining data protection, and clarifying liability issues. The integration of clinical research and medical practice necessitates clear guidelines to protect patients' rights while maximizing the potential of AI. At the same time, AI is fundamentally changing healthcare delivery, placing new demands on specialists and existing infrastructures. Future regulations must therefore provide legal certainty and promote innovation while consistently ensuring transparency, fairness, and patient protection.

Introduction

The healthcare industry is undergoing a fundamental transformation driven by AI integration. AI-powered systems enable the analysis of large-scale medical data, assist healthcare professionals in diagnostics and therapy planning, and improve patient care. In radiology, AI algorithms can accelerate the detection of suspicious tumor structures, often surpassing human capabilities in speed and accuracy. Similarly, in personalized medicine, AI plays a crucial role in developing customized therapeutic interventions. At the same time, AI utilization raises significant ethical concerns, including the transparency and interpretability of AI decisions and the legal implications of incorrect diagnoses. Additionally, there is a need to address the tension between strict data protection requirements and the necessity for large datasets to train AI models.

To address these challenges, different countries are implementing varied regulatory approaches. The European Union (EU) has adopted a preventive, risk-based strategy through the AI Act, the MDR, and the GDPR, placing significant emphasis on transparency, security, and data protection. Conversely, the United States (US) has opted for a more sector-specific and flexible regulatory framework, which, while promoting innovation, also introduces regulatory uncertainty. These contrasting regulatory landscapes have far-reaching implications for AI systems' market access and the safeguarding of patient rights.

This chapter first examines the legal and ethical challenges associated with AI use in healthcare (section "Ethical and Legal Challenges of the Use of AI in the Healthcare Sector"). It then analyzes the regulatory framework in the EU (section "Regulatory Framework Conditions in the EU") and the US (section "Regulatory Framework in the USA"), followed by a comparison of the two approaches (section "Comparison of Regulatory Approaches and Remaining Challenges"). Finally, an outlook on future developments is provided (section "Outlook and Conclusions").

The aim is to enhance the understanding of regulatory requirements and illustrate how legal certainty, innovation promotion, and patient protection can be effectively balanced.

Ethical and Legal Challenges of the Use of AI in the Healthcare Sector

The growing integration of artificial intelligence (AI) is fundamentally transforming the healthcare sector. AI assists professionals with diagnostics, therapy planning, patient monitoring, and care by processing large volumes of data and providing evidence-based recommendations. At the same time, its use raises numerous ethical and legal concerns.

Transparency and Informed Consent

A key challenge in the use of AI in healthcare is the lack of transparency in many systems, which can compromise patient autonomy and the principle of informed consent. Traditionally, every medical decision relies on patients making autonomous choices about their treatment after being fully informed about the benefits, risks, and alternatives. The growing use of AI introduces new challenges to this principle.

Many AI applications, especially those based on deep learning, function as "black boxes", making them difficult to interpret. If even healthcare professionals struggle to understand how an AI system reaches its decisions, it becomes nearly impossible for patients to make informed choices. This may lead them to passively accept AI recommendations without questioning them. As a result, non-transparent systems not only create uncertainty among healthcare professionals but also restrict patients' freedom of choice.

This issue is particularly concerning for adaptive AI systems, which continuously evolve. While traditional medical devices or software remain unchanged after approval, modern AI models can modify their decision-making processes by integrating new data. This raises the question of whether informed consent, once given, remains valid. If assessment patterns shift, it is unclear whether patients would provide consent again under comparable conditions.

The lack of explainability in AI decisions is therefore not only an ethical issue but also a legal one. Informed consent requires that patients comprehend what they are agreeing to. If AI decision-making processes lack sufficient transparency, this fundamental requirement is undermined. Ultimately, a lack of transparency not only limits patients' freedom of choice but may also jeopardize legal certainty.

Bias and Fair Decision-Making

Bias and structural inequalities present a major challenge in the use of AI in healthcare. The reliability of medical AI systems heavily depends on the quality of the data used for training. However, such data often reflects existing social and medical disparities, which can be embedded into the algorithms. Studies have shown, for example, that AI-assisted skin cancer diagnoses are less accurate for individuals with darker skin tones and that algorithms used in emergency rooms may unintentionally reinforce social inequalities.

If biases in training data are not actively identified and corrected, there is a risk that certain patient groups will face systematic disadvantages. Therefore, the development and application of medical AI systems must ensure that algorithms do not perpetuate discriminatory patterns. This issue is particularly critical, as biases can impact not only individual diagnostic accuracy but also scientific research and data-driven medical advancements. If AI models are primarily trained on data from specific population groups, there is a risk that research findings will lack generalizability, leading to disparities in treatment outcomes.

Liability for AI-Supported Decisions

The introduction of AI systems into healthcare not only transforms workflows but also redefines liability allocation. Traditionally, responsibility has rested with doctors and other medical professionals who make treatment decisions. However, the use of AI introduces legal uncertainties, particularly when algorithms generate erroneous diagnoses or treatment recommendations based on flawed or biased training data.

Medical professionals remain responsible for critically evaluating AI-supported recommendations. Simultaneously, manufacturers and healthcare facilities are accountable for the reliability of these systems and must ensure they do not produce inaccurate or non-transparent decisions. Beyond initial regulatory approval, continuous monitoring and adaptation are required. This challenge is particularly pronounced in the case of adaptive AI systems that evolve after market introduction. It remains unclear whether liability for incorrect diagnoses lies with medical staff, healthcare institutions, or the manufacturer. In the absence of clear legal guidelines, such ambiguities create obstacles for both the practical implementation and further advancement of AI-driven healthcare solutions.

AI and the Role of the Healthcare Professions

The integration of AI systems not only transforms workflows but also redefines the role of healthcare professionals. As AI technologies increasingly assist in decision-making, clinicians' responsibilities shift toward evaluating AI-generated recommendations and contextualizing them within clinical practice. This evolution introduces new demands for training and professional practice.

Beyond technical expertise, proficiency in AI utilization is becoming a critical skill. Healthcare professionals must grasp how algorithms function, critically assess their outputs, and effectively incorporate them into interdisciplinary decision-making processes. Additionally, the implementation of AI necessitates enhanced collaboration among physicians, nurses, and other healthcare professionals, as AI-driven systems operate within interconnected domains of patient care rather than in isolation.

Technology and Patient Interaction

The growing use of AI in the healthcare sector not only alters diagnostic and therapeutic processes but also reshapes the interaction between healthcare professionals and patients. Personal relationships remain fundamental, particularly in nursing and medical care. The increasing reliance on AI-driven assistance systems and robotics can impact interpersonal communication, especially when routine tasks are automated, or AI systems propose treatment decisions.

However, patients expect more than precise medical assessments and optimal treatment—they also seek personalized attention and compassionate care. Thus, the responsible use of AI must strike a balance between technological support and human empathy.

Data Protection and Research

The application of AI in healthcare relies on large volumes of patient data, utilized both for personalized treatment and medical research. However, the distinction between clinical care and data-driven research is becoming increasingly blurred. Many AI systems not only rely on historical data sets but also evolve through continuous application. This raises ethical and data protection concerns, particularly when patient data is used to refine algorithms without explicit consent.

A key issue is that patients are often unaware that their health data may be utilized not only for their own treatment but also for research purposes. While insights from clinical data advance medical procedures, such use must respect informational self-determination. Additionally, it remains unclear to what extent previously collected data may be repurposed for future AI-driven analyses, particularly as algorithms continuously evolve.

Modern AI models demand extensive and diverse data sets to achieve reliability. Simultaneously, strict data protection laws limit the collection and use of personal data, creating a conflict between the need for high-quality training data and the obligation to uphold data privacy. This challenge intensifies in international research projects, where cross-border data sharing is subject to additional legal constraints.

Balancing data protection requirements with the needs of data-driven research and clinical practice remains one of AI's greatest challenges in healthcare. Addressing this requires clear regulations and transparent procedures that safeguard patient data while supporting the advancement of innovative AI applications.

Regulatory Framework Conditions in the EU

The regulation of AI use in the European healthcare sector relies on three pillars: two general regulatory frameworks with cross-industry applicability and a sector-specific regulation for medical devices.

The first general pillar is the AI Act, which introduces uniform regulations for AI for the first time. It establishes requirements for safety, transparency, and risk management, covering both medical and non-medical applications. The second general pillar is the General Data Protection Regulation (GDPR), which ensures that personal health data is processed only under strict data protection requirements.

The third pillar is the Medical Device Regulation (MDR), a sector-specific framework that determines when AI applications qualify as medical devices and specifies the necessary safety and performance standards. Complementing these binding regulations, the European Commission has issued ethical guidelines for trustworthy AI. Although not legally binding, these guidelines establish best practices for the responsible development and use of AI, emphasizing core principles such as fairness, transparency, and human-centric AI design.

AI Act: Risk-Based Regulation of AI

The Artificial Intelligence Act (AI Act) is the first comprehensive regulatory framework for artificial intelligence in the European Union (EU). While the MDR establishes specific requirements for AI-powered medical devices, the AI Act applies across all sectors, including healthcare. Its primary goal is to classify AI systems based on their risk potential and define appropriate regulatory obligations accordingly.

The AI Act follows a risk-based approach, categorizing AI systems into four levels—ranging from minimal risk to high-risk applications. Most AI systems in healthcare fall under the high-risk category, particularly when they assist in diagnoses, influence treatment decisions, or actively intervene in medical processes. For such systems, the AI Act mandates strict requirements for traceability, transparency, and accountability.

A key focus of the AI Act is the explainability of AI-generated decisions. Medical professionals must be able to understand the reasoning behind AI-generated diagnoses or treatment recommendations. This ensures that medical decisions do not rely on unverifiable or opaque algorithms.

Another essential component of the AI Act is the mitigation of bias and prevention of discrimination. Developers are required to ensure that training data is diverse, representative, and robust. Without proactive bias detection and correction, certain patient groups may face systematic disadvantages, and AI-driven diagnoses may be unreliable. The regulation, therefore, mandates mechanisms for bias detection, reduction, and regular validation of training datasets.

Particularly stringent requirements apply to adaptive and self-learning AI models that evolve after market introduction. The AI Act requires that high-risk AI systems remain under human oversight and do not undergo uncontrolled modifications. Medical professionals must be empowered to review, adjust, or override AI-supported diagnoses or treatment recommendations. This safeguard aims to prevent over-reliance on AI, which could result in incorrect clinical decisions.

The AI Act's provisions will be implemented gradually starting in 2026, allowing companies and healthcare institutions sufficient time to comply. However, the AI Act is already recognized as a cornerstone of AI regulation in the EU, as it not only establishes legal obligations but also promotes a unified European strategy for the trustworthy and responsible use of AI in healthcare.

GDPR: Requirements for the Handling of Health Data

The GDPR constitutes the second general pillar of AI regulation in the European Union (EU). While the AI Act establishes broad requirements for safety, reliability, transparency, and risk management, the GDPR governs the conditions under which personal data may be processed. Since medical AI applications rely heavily on sensitive health data, GDPR compliance is crucial for developers, healthcare providers, and research institutions.

Article 9 of the GDPR classifies health data as a specially protected category of personal data, restricting processing unless explicit, informed, and voluntary consent is obtained or a legal exemption applies. In practice, AI applications in healthcare must either secure individual consent or operate under a legally defined basis. The GDPR mandates that patients fully understand what data is being processed, for what purpose, and with what implications. This ensures strict data protection standards.

Additionally, the GDPR shapes the technical design of AI systems through several core data protection principles. The principle of purpose limitation restricts data use to clearly defined and legitimate purposes. This poses challenges if AI models need to expand beyond their initial scope or be retrained with new datasets. The principle of data minimization requires processing only essential data, which can conflict with the need for large, diverse datasets in AI training. Another key requirement is transparency—data controllers must inform individuals about how and why their data is processed, particularly in automated decision-making. This is especially complex for deep learning-based AI systems, where decision-making processes are often difficult to interpret.

Healthcare practitioners must navigate the tension between data protection laws and AI's technical requirements. To comply with GDPR, they employ pseudonymization and anonymization to preserve data privacy without compromising AI training quality.

The GDPR also imposes strict requirements on transferring personal data to third countries. Personal data from EU citizens may only be shared with nations like the USA if an adequate level of protection is ensured. This prevents weakened data protection standards through processing abroad. These rules are particularly critical for international research collaborations, as they significantly limit the exchange of medical data with non-EU partners.

MDR: Requirements for AI-Supported Medical Devices

The Medical Device Regulation (MDR) serves as the sector-specific pillar of European AI regulation in healthcare, complementing the general requirements of the AI Act and the GDPR. While these two regulations apply to AI applications across various sectors, the MDR establishes specific requirements for AI-powered medical devices. It defines when an AI system qualifies as a medical device and outlines the regulatory standards it must meet. This is particularly relevant for applications in diagnostics, therapy planning, and patient monitoring.

The MDR adopts a risk-based approach, categorizing AI-based medical devices into three classes based on their potential risk and clinical significance. Class I devices, which pose low risk, include simple software applications used for administrative purposes and are subject to minimal regulatory requirements. Medium-to-high-risk systems, classified as IIa and IIb, cover AI-powered solutions for diagnostic support, therapy planning, and patient monitoring. These require more extensive regulatory scrutiny, as they directly impact patient care. Class III, representing high-risk AI applications, includes systems that make independent medical decisions or actively intervene in treatment processes, such as surgical assistance systems or intelligent monitoring solutions for intensive care patients. These systems must undergo a comprehensive clinical evaluation before receiving approval.

Regardless of the risk classification, manufacturers must demonstrate the safety and effectiveness of their AI systems. This involves providing detailed technical documentation describing functionality and safety measures, conducting a clinical evaluation to verify the system's reliability and effectiveness in real-world medical settings, and implementing risk management protocols to identify potential hazards and introduce appropriate risk-mitigation measures. While Class I devices can often enter the market through a self-declaration by the manufacturer, products in Class IIa and above require a conformity assessment by a notified body. These external inspection bodies, accredited by regulatory authorities, evaluate compliance with MDR requirements.

A post-market surveillance system (PMS) is mandatory to ensure the continued safety and performance of AI-powered medical devices after their market launch.

This is particularly critical for adaptive AI systems, which evolve through continuous learning. The MDR imposes strict requirements on post-market monitoring for such systems. AI applications that continue learning after deployment must remain in compliance with regulatory standards, necessitating ongoing testing mechanisms to assess performance and safety and regular reassessments if the AI undergoes significant modifications. As the risk level of an AI-powered medical device increases, so do the requirements for continuous monitoring and regulatory oversight.

Ethical Guidelines for AI in the EU

In addition to the binding requirements of the AI Act, GDPR, and MDR, the EU has established ethical guidelines for trustworthy AI. While not legally binding, these guidelines set best practices for AI development and use in healthcare. Whereas legal regulations focus on technical and legal compliance, ethical guidelines emphasize social and moral aspects of AI applications.

A core principle is human-centric AI design—AI should support rather than replace healthcare professionals. The AI Act prohibits autonomous decision-making in high-risk AI, but ethics guidelines go further, stressing that AI must not create dependency or reduce medical staff responsibility.

Another key focus is fairness and non-discrimination. Bias in training data can disadvantage certain patient groups or lead to incorrect diagnoses. While the AI Act mandates bias-reduction measures, ethics guidelines advocate ongoing ethical reviews to detect discrimination early and promote equal access to AI-driven healthcare.

Closely linked is the principle of accountability. The AI Act assigns clear responsibilities for high-risk AI, and the GDPR regulates data protection, but ethics guidelines address practical liability issues, especially for unexpected risks or incorrect decisions.

Data protection and transparency also play a central role. The GDPR mandates strict data protection, while the AI Act requires transparency and traceability. Ethics guidelines go beyond legal compliance, emphasizing the importance of patient trust in AI-driven healthcare. Clear communication should inform patients how AI influences their treatment and what choices remain under their control.

Although not legally binding, ethical guidelines shape regulatory developments and serve as a framework for responsible AI use in healthcare. Many European companies voluntarily follow the Assessment List for Trustworthy AI (ALTAI) or participate in the EU AI Alliance to implement ethical standards and foster trust in AI technologies.

Regulatory Framework in the USA

Unlike the European Union, which has established a structured AI regulation in healthcare through the AI Act and GDPR as general frameworks and the MDR as a sector-specific regulation, the United States follow a decentralized, sector-based approach. There is no nationwide AI legislation; instead, regulatory requirements stem from medical device law, data protection law, and liability law, which vary in interpretation and enforcement across federal agencies and individual states.

Medical Device Regulations and the Role of the FDA

The U.S. Food and Drug Administration (FDA) serves as the primary regulatory authority for AI-driven applications in healthcare. It oversees the approval and monitoring of Software as a Medical Device (SaMD) and Software in a Medical Device (SiMD). SaMD includes stand-alone AI applications, such as diagnostic algorithms and therapy planning tools, while SiMD refers to software integrated into physical medical devices, such as imaging systems or surgical assistance technologies.

Similar to the EU's risk-based classification, the FDA categorizes AI-supported medical devices based on potential risk and clinical significance, subjecting them to different levels of regulatory scrutiny. Low-risk applications, such as administrative hospital software, must only meet general regulatory standards. In contrast, higher-risk systems that assist in diagnosis or influence treatment decisions require formal regulatory approval. High-risk AI, including early cancer detection algorithms and surgical assistance systems, undergoes particularly rigorous testing.

A major difference from the EU's AI Act concerns adaptive AI models. While the AI Act mandates continuous validation of learning systems, the FDA follows a more flexible approach with its Predetermined Change Control Plan. This allows manufacturers to pre-register planned modifications, enabling post-approval algorithm updates without requiring a full regulatory review for each change. While this accelerates AI system development, it also raises concerns about long-term oversight and traceability of AI decisions.

Ongoing regulatory initiatives under the current U.S. administration may lead to revisions of FDA requirements, particularly regarding potentially more flexible approval processes for AI-driven medical devices.

Data Protection Framework Conditions

Unlike the EU, which has established a uniform data protection framework under the GDPR, the U.S. legal landscape consists of a patchwork of federal and state-level regulations.

Health data protection in the U.S. is primarily governed by the Health Insurance Portability and Accountability Act (HIPAA), which regulates the handling of Protected Health Information (PHI). HIPAA mandates that hospitals, insurers, and other healthcare providers implement specific data protection measures. However, HIPAA applies only to "Covered Entities", meaning many AI developers and technology companies—such as those offering health apps, wearables (e.g., fitness trackers), or AI-driven diagnostic tools—are not subject to HIPAA's provisions. Companies that do not directly collaborate with healthcare providers or insurers therefore operate outside a uniform regulatory framework.

A key difference between HIPAA and the GDPR lies in purpose limitation. While both frameworks permit the processing of health data for treatment and research, they impose different conditions. The GDPR mandates strict protective measures, such as transparency obligations, pseudonymization, and explicit purpose limitation. In contrast, HIPAA allows broader and more flexible data use, enabling health data to be leveraged for AI model development or medical service optimization without the same level of restrictions as in the EU.

Recent political discussions in the U.S. suggest a potential revision of data protection laws, which could impact HIPAA and patient data protection. While the GDPR enforces strict purpose limitation in the EU, the U.S. approach prioritizes flexibility, particularly in the context of AI-driven innovation.

Additionally, state-level laws—such as the California Consumer Privacy Act (CCPA) and the California Privacy Rights Act (CPRA)—grant consumers greater rights, particularly regarding data transparency and control. However, these regulations apply only to businesses operating in California, leading to an inconsistent data protection landscape across the U.S.

Ethical Guidelines and Voluntary Self-Regulation

In the European Union, the ethical guidelines for trustworthy AI complement legal regulations by providing an overarching ethical framework. In contrast, the United States lacks a central, binding AI ethics framework. Instead, various institutions have issued non-binding guidelines.

One of the most notable initiatives is the AI Risk Management Framework developed by the National Institute of Standards and Technology (NIST). This framework offers recommendations on fairness, transparency, and security, but does not carry legal weight. Additionally, the Biden administration had introduced the Blueprint for an AI Bill of Rights, which should promote human-centric AI principles, including data protection, security, and non-discrimination. However, this blueprint had served only as guidance and does not create legal obligations for businesses or regulatory agencies.

Beyond government initiatives, many technology companies and healthcare institutions have established their own AI ethics policies. For instance, Microsoft has developed internal guidelines emphasizing transparency, accountability, and inclusion in AI development. However, such corporate policies vary widely, as companies determine independently which ethical principles to follow and how to enforce them.

Comparison of Regulatory Approaches and Remaining Challenges

The regulation of artificial intelligence (AI) in healthcare differs significantly between the European Union (EU) and the United States (US) in both structural approach and substantive focus. While the EU follows a preventive, risk-based regulatory framework, the US adopts a sector-specific, flexible, and market-driven approach. Each model has its strengths but also leaves regulatory gaps that impact practical implementation (Table 11.1).

Regulatory Approach: Uniformity Versus Flexibility

The EU's AI regulatory framework, shaped by the AI Act, the Medical Device Regulation (MDR), and the General Data Protection Regulation (GDPR), combines clear legal requirements with centralized oversight by European institutions. This preventive approach ensures that AI applications meet strict safety, transparency, and data protection requirements before they are deployed. The classification of high-risk AI systems allows for proactive oversight, helping to identify risks early and prevent harmful developments.

In contrast, the US lacks a unified AI regulation. Instead, existing laws and agencies govern AI, with the Food and Drug Administration (FDA) overseeing medical devices and the Health Insurance Portability and Accountability Act (HIPAA)

Table 11.1 Comparison of AI healthcare regulations: EU vs. USA

Category	EU approach	US approach
Regulatory approach	Preventive, risk-based regulations (AI Act, MDR, GDPR)	Sector specific, market driven (FDA, HIPAA)
Data protection and processing	Strict data protection (GDPR: Data minimization, purpose limitation)	Fragmented, flexible (HIPAA applies only to "covered entities"
Medical device regulation	MDR: Strict safety testing and risk classification	FDA: Post-market flexibility, rapid adaption
Liability for AI decisions	Manufacturers liable for high-risk AI, unclear for evolving AI	Doctors/hospitals liable for AI errors; manufacturers only for clear defects
Ethics and transparency	Mandatory transparency and explainability for high-risk AI	No legal transparency mandate, voluntary industry self-regulation

regulating health data privacy. This industry-specific and reactive approach means that AI regulations are often updated after new technologies have already entered the market.

These regulatory differences directly influence innovation speed. In the EU, companies must navigate a rigorous compliance process before an AI system receives approval. The US's more flexible system allows for faster development and deployment. This speed, however, comes at the cost of greater uncertainty for patients, healthcare providers, and regulators, as there are no consistent requirements for transparency, bias mitigation, or long-term monitoring of adaptive AI systems.

Data Protection and Data Processing: Strict Requirements Versus Flexible Use

A major difference between the EU and the US lies in the regulation of health data. The GDPR imposes strict requirements on the processing of personal health data, particularly through the principles of data minimization and purpose limitation. While these measures provide strong patient protection, they also pose challenges for the development of AI systems, which require large datasets for training.

In contrast, the US follows a less restrictive yet fragmented approach under HIPAA. Companies have greater flexibility in using health data for research and development, provided they comply with HIPAA regulations. However, HIPAA applies only to "covered entities", such as hospitals, insurers, and healthcare providers, meaning that many technology companies processing health data are not subject to this law. As a result, data protection standards vary depending on the actor and intended use, leading to inconsistencies in regulation.

Another challenge is the international exchange of health data. While the GDPR ensures a uniform level of protection within the EU, the US and other countries have divergent data protection requirements, complicating cross-border medical data sharing for research. Additionally, GDPR opening clauses allow EU member states to implement supplementary regulations, leading to further discrepancies and hindering full regulatory harmonization. These differences negatively impact the development of AI-driven healthcare applications, as many AI models rely on broad, diverse, and interoperable datasets.

Regulation of AI-Supported Medical Devices: Strict Requirements Versus Post-Regulation

In the EU, AI-based medical devices are regulated under the MDR, which establishes strict requirements for safety testing and risk classification. Depending on their risk category, AI systems must undergo a conformity assessment and, if required, be evaluated by notified bodies. High-risk AI applications, such as AI-assisted surgical systems, are subject to particularly rigorous requirements to ensure patient safety and clinical reliability.

In contrast, the US regulates AI-based medical devices through the FDA, which classifies them as "Software as a Medical Device" (SaMD). The FDA's approach is more flexible, allowing AI models to evolve post-market without requiring full re-approval. While this accelerates innovation, it also creates regulatory gray areas, particularly when an AI system undergoes substantial changes through self-learning mechanisms after its approval. The AI Act in the EU strictly regulates such adaptive systems, imposing clear traceability and oversight requirements, whereas the FDA's framework prioritizes flexibility, benefiting manufacturers but potentially reducing transparency for users.

Liability for AI Decisions

Liability for incorrect AI-driven decisions remains a major regulatory challenge in both the EU and the USA.

In the European Union, primary liability rests with manufacturers of high-risk AI, who are responsible for ensuring safety and regulatory compliance under the AI Act and MDR. However, doctors and healthcare providers also bear legal responsibility for using AI-assisted systems. A key uncertainty is the extent to which clinicians must independently verify AI-generated recommendations or whether they can rely on them. The issue is particularly complex for self-learning AI models—if an AI alters its decision-making processes post-market, it remains unclear whether re-certification is required.

In the United States, there is no specific AI liability regulation. Instead, liability is governed by general product liability laws and medical malpractice principles. In practice, this means that doctors are primarily liable if they adopt an incorrect AI recommendation, while manufacturers are only held accountable if a clear product defect can be demonstrated.

A key difference between the EU and the USA is the treatment of adaptive AI. Under the Predetermined Change Control Plan, the FDA allows manufacturers to update AI models after approval without requiring a full re-evaluation for each change. While this accelerates innovation, it also raises concerns about long-term oversight, as an approved AI may change its decision-making processes without undergoing a new regulatory review.

Ethics and Transparency: Different Approaches to Building Trust

The EU places strong emphasis on ethical principles, particularly through the ethical guidelines for trustworthy AI and mandatory transparency and explainability requirements for high-risk AI. These measures aim to ensure that medical decisions are understandable and fair.

In contrast, the USA relies more on private-sector self-regulation. There is no legal obligation for AI algorithms to be transparent, allowing companies to decide how much they disclose about their systems. This can lead to trust issues, especially when patients and healthcare providers cannot fully understand how an AI system generates diagnoses or treatment recommendations. While the AI Act mandates human-centered AI, the implementation of ethical principles in the USA remains largely voluntary and dependent on corporate commitments.

Conclusion

The regulation of AI in healthcare reveals clear differences between the EU and the USA. While the EU follows a preventive and uniform framework, the US allows for a more flexible, sector-specific approach. Both models have advantages and disadvantages, making the debate over the optimal regulatory approach an ongoing issue in both policy and scientific discussion.

Outlook and Conclusions

The regulation of artificial intelligence in healthcare is an ongoing process that must adapt to technological, social, and political developments. This dynamic landscape presents major challenges for existing regulatory frameworks. While the European Union has established a comprehensive but complex regulatory structure through the AI Act, MDR, and GDPR, the United States follows a more fragmented and adaptable approach. Over the next few years, it will become clear whether these regulatory models can keep pace with the rapid evolution of AI technologies or whether further adjustments will be necessary. Regulatory frameworks must strike a balance between legal certainty and fostering innovation to ensure that AI develops in a safe and effective manner.

The regulation of adaptive and self-learning AI systems will remain a key area of concern. In the EU, uncertainty persists regarding how much an approved AI system can evolve before requiring recertification. While the AI Act mandates transparency and traceability, practical implementation challenges remain. The US approach places greater responsibility on manufacturers, allowing faster adaptation to technological advancements but also creating regulatory gray areas. The challenge will be to develop mechanisms that allow AI systems to evolve while maintaining clear oversight. One possible solution could be regulatory “sandboxes”, where new AI technologies can be tested under controlled conditions before receiving final market approval.

Further development of regulation is also likely to be necessary in the area of data protection. While the GDPR sets strict requirements for the use of large health data sets further regulatory developments are likely to be necessary in data protection. The GDPR imposes strict requirements on the use of large health data sets through purpose limitation and data minimization, thereby restricting AI model training, the less restrictive data protection laws in the USA provide greater flexibility for developing data-driven technologies. Additionally, national opening clauses within the EU create further fragmentation. Although the GDPR was designed to establish uniform data protection standards, in practice, member states impose varying requirements on medical data processing due to national exemptions. As a result, AI companies and research institutions in some EU countries have easier access to health data than in others, making cross-border AI deployment more complex. In contrast, HIPAA in the US applies only to specific entities, meaning that many technology companies are not subject to the same data protection obligations. Greater international coordination could help safeguard sensitive patient data while facilitating health data research.

Regulation must also address the growing tension between data protection requirements and data-driven innovation. While the GDPR imposes strict limitations on large-scale health data use for AI training, US regulations offer more flexibility. This also affects transatlantic data exchange: European entities must comply with strict GDPR rules, while the US lacks an equivalent comprehensive data protection framework. The legal discrepancies not only hinder cross-border medical data exchange for research and development but could also disadvantage European companies in global competition. Finding solutions that ensure data protection without hindering medical progress will be critical.

These regulatory differences impact not only data protection but also innovation speed. While the GDPR provides legal certainty, its strict requirements make it challenging to use health data for AI development. In contrast, US companies benefit from greater flexibility but must navigate a fragmented regulatory environment. As AI increasingly relies on large, diverse data sets, the pressure on legislators will grow to strike a balance between data protection and enabling data-driven research.

Technological advancements will continue to introduce new regulatory challenges. Explainable AI (XAI) is becoming increasingly important as it supports regulatory compliance with requirements for accountability and patient education. Additionally, federated learning and privacy-preserving AI models offer potential solutions for leveraging large health datasets while complying with privacy regulations. However, AI-driven personalized medicine presents new obstacles for existing regulatory frameworks, particularly when systems continuously adapt based on individual patient data, which may conflict with traditional approval processes.

Beyond technological and regulatory considerations, the integration of AI into everyday clinical practice must be addressed. The adoption of AI in healthcare is reshaping professional roles, affecting medical responsibility, data transparency, and informed consent. Additionally, growing dependence on data-driven processes is blurring the lines between clinical research and algorithmic decision-making, potentially transforming how medical innovations are developed and validated.

At the same time, the intersection of clinical research and data-driven AI research is strengthening. AI models rely increasingly on vast health datasets to refine diagnostic and therapeutic capabilities, which challenges existing ethical and regulatory frameworks. Distinguishing between patient data usage for direct treatment versus scientific or commercial purposes becomes crucial. Without clear regulatory guidelines, healthcare professionals risk passively endorsing AI decisions without fully scrutinizing them, while patients may unknowingly become part of research processes without understanding the implications. Future regulatory strategies must ensure that AI enhances medical decision-making while enabling patients to make informed choices, without compromising ethical principle.

Beyond national regulations, global harmonization is becoming increasingly important. Divergent regulatory requirements in the EU, USA, China, and Japan complicate the development and deployment of globally applicable AI solutions. Establishing uniform standards for safety, transparency, and data quality would facilitate market access for innovative healthcare applications. While the EU has taken the lead with the AI Act, a lack of equivalent international guidelines hinders parallel approvals across multiple jurisdictions. Whether common global standards emerge will depend on political and economic cooperation among major economic blocs.

In the long run, it remains to be seen whether a sustainable balance between innovation and patient protection can be achieved. Targeted regulation that integrates ethical principles into technological development will be crucial in determining whether AI reaches its full potential in healthcare. A key priority will be ensuring that AI decision-making processes are transparent, comprehensible, and trustworthy, preventing bias and discrimination.

For the EU, greater coordination between the AI Act, MDR, and GDPR may be necessary to reduce regulatory overlaps and contradictions. In particular, adapting data protection regulations to learning AI systems could become a central focus of future regulatory developments—especially concerning purpose limitation and the subsequent use of health data.

In the USA, there are ongoing discussions on further developing AI regulations, but it remains unclear whether future initiatives will lead to greater standardization at the federal level or if the current fragmented sectoral approach will continue.

Overall, AI regulation in healthcare remains a dynamic and evolving field that requires continuous adaptation. The key challenge will be how lawmakers in both regions manage the delicate balance between fostering innovation and ensuring patient safety. Stronger international dialogue on regulatory best practices could help establish more globally consistent and innovation-friendly frameworks.

The coming years will present new regulatory challenges and well-designed policies will play a crucial role in maximizing AI's potential in healthcare—all while maintaining the highest ethical and safety standards.

Useful Resources

Overview of the regulatory landscape for artificial intelligence in health within the European Union. https://www.nature.com/articles/s41746-024-01221-6

From Soft Law to Hard Choices: Healthcare AI Governance Across the USA and EU. https://irpj.euclid.int/articles/from-soft-law-to-hard-choices-healthcare-ai-governance-across-the-usa-and-eu/

Regulierung von KI in den USA. https://www.gtai.de/de/trade/usa/recht/regulierung-von-ki-in-den-usa-1832964

Navigating the European Union Artificial Intelligence Act for Healthcare. https://www.nature.com/articles/s41746-024-01213-6

Legal and Ethical Consideration in Artificial Intelligence in Healthcare: Who Takes Responsibility? https://www.frontiersin.org/journals/surgery/articles/10.3389/fsurg.2022.862322/full

Global Regulatory Frameworks for the Use of Artificial Intelligence in Healthcare. https://pmc.ncbi.nlm.nih.gov/articles/PMC10930608/

Digital Innovations in Healthcare. https://osnadocs.ub.uni-osnabrueck.de/bitstream/ds-2023120810135/9/thesis_arlinghaus.pdf

Artificial Intelligence Regulatory Resource Guide. https://www.ahima.org/media/twjmtnq4/2024-artificial-intelligence-regulatory-resource-guide-axs.pdf

Review Questions

1. What are the key differences between the EU and US approaches to regulating AI in healthcare, and what challenges do these frameworks create for companies, clinicians, and patients?
2. How does bias in AI-based diagnosis and treatment recommendations pose risks, and what regulatory measures exist to prevent discriminatory algorithms?
3. What challenges does AI pose for informed consent in medical diagnosis, particularly in terms of algorithmic transparency and traceability?
4. To what extent can ethical guidelines complement or substitute existing legal frameworks for AI regulation in healthcare?
5. What regulatory approaches could better balance innovation, liability concerns, and the protection of patient data in the future?
6. How do the EU and US differ in their approaches to liability for AI-based medical decisions, and what challenges does this create for healthcare providers and developers?

Answers to Review Questions

1. The EU regulates AI in healthcare through the AI Act, MDR, and GDPR, focusing on preventive, industry-specific rules with strict transparency, security, and data protection requirements. This ensures legal clarity for patients and clinics but may slow innovation. The US follows a more flexible, sector-based approach, with fragmented regulation by the FDA and HIPAA. While this facilitates faster

market entry for AI products, it creates regulatory uncertainty and weaker data protection. The EU model offers greater legal certainty, whereas the US framework allows for quicker innovation but raises concerns about patient rights and inconsistent application.

2. Bias in AI can lead to unequal treatment and incorrect diagnoses. The EU requires manufacturers to assess training data for bias and implement measures against discrimination. In contrast, the US imposes fewer mandatory requirements, relying instead on voluntary industry standards.
3. Many AI models, particularly self-learning systems, lack transparency, making it difficult for patients to make informed decisions. The EU mandates explainable AI, but implementing this effectively remains challenging, especially for systems that evolve after deployment.
4. Ethical guidelines provide essential standards for fairness, transparency, and accountability. While they complement legal frameworks by offering guidance where laws are unclear, they cannot replace binding regulations, as they are not legally enforceable.
5. Regulatory "sandboxes" could enable real-world testing of AI innovations without requiring full regulatory compliance from the outset. Clearer liability frameworks for adaptive AI systems and stronger international coordination could also help balance innovation with legal certainty and data protection.
6. Liability for AI-driven medical decisions varies significantly between the EU and the US. In the EU, manufacturers bear primary responsibility for high-risk AI under the AI Act and MDR, while medical professionals must review AI recommendations. However, liability remains unclear if a self-learning AI alters its decision-making after market launch. The US lacks specific AI liability laws, meaning doctors and clinics are generally liable for incorrect AI-based decisions, while manufacturers are only accountable for proven product defects. The EU offers greater legal certainty through clear manufacturer responsibility, whereas the US approach fosters innovation but leaves liability questions unresolved.

Chapter 12
Ethical Theories for Artificial Intelligence (AI) in Healthcare

David L. Meyers and Emily Grime

Learning Objectives

- To identify and explain Ethical Theories and Frameworks for evaluation and decision-making: Students will learn and understand major ethical theories, such as utilitarianism, deontology, virtue ethics and other approaches to explain how they can be applied to ethical questions and challenges posed by AI technologies in healthcare.
- To evaluate and resolve ethical dilemmas: Students will consider specific ethical questions and dilemmas related to the use of AI in healthcare, utilizing various ethical approaches to evaluate potential solutions and outcomes.
- To evaluate AI's impact on various aspects of health care: Students will evaluate the implications of AI technologies on patient care, research, education and other areas with respect to equity, privacy, consent, and other relevant features through the lenses of different ethical frameworks.
- To discuss accountability and responsibility: Students will discuss the concepts of accountability and responsibility in the context of AI decision-making in healthcare, articulating how ethical theories inform the roles and practices of healthcare professionals—clinicians, researchers, educators and other health care workers, developers, institutions, communities and the larger society.
- To develop Ethical Guidelines: Students will be able to develop a set of ethical guidelines or recommendations for the implementation of AI in healthcare settings, integrating insights from ethical theories to ensure patient-centered and ethically sound practices.

D. L. Meyers (✉)
Mount Washington, MD, USA

E. Grime
Tampa, FL, USA

U. H. Hübner et al. (eds.), *Bridging Artificial and Human Intelligence*, Health Informatics, https://doi.org/10.1007/978-3-032-11938-4_12

Key Terms

- Morality
- Common Morality
- Utilitarianism
- Deontology
- Virtue Ethics
- Informed Consent
- Bias and Fairness
- Principlism which includes
  - Beneficence
  - Non-Maleficence
  - Justice
  - Autonomy

Summary

This chapter explores the intersection of ethical frameworks and the deployment of artificial intelligence (AI) in healthcare, addressing the complexities and challenges posed by technological advancements. It begins by outlining fundamental ethical theories and principles which offer frameworks for ethical decision-making in the context of AI.

Specific ethical dilemmas that arise from the integration of AI in healthcare, such as patient autonomy, informed consent, bias in algorithmic decision-making and others will be examined. Through the lenses of these ethical frameworks, various scenarios where AI technologies may impact elements of healthcare and stakeholders will be presented in order to arrive at ethical conclusions in decision-making.

Key discussions will focus on the necessity of establishing ethical guidelines that prioritize patient welfare and equity and facilitate decision-making in all categories of healthcare stakeholders—patients, clinicians, administrators, health informatics workers, AI developers, researchers, educators, regulators—and across the various corporate enterprises involved in health services and products. These guidelines must ensure accountability for all AI-driven decisions. The chapter emphasizes the importance of fostering a patient-centered approach, advocating for fairness and transparency in AI applications.

Introduction

The rapid advancement of AI is transforming the entire landscape of healthcare and clinical practice, showing promise in enhancing diagnostic accuracy, personalizing treatment plans, influencing the development of therapeutics and technologies, guiding research and professional education, streamlining administrative processes and even creating scripts for difficult conversations [1]. This raises profound ethical questions which must be understood to ensure that the best interests of patients and society are served. Exploring the major ethical theories and decisional frameworks, including utilitarianism, deontology, virtue ethics and principlism, will provide approaches for addressing these challenges.

Ethics Concepts and Theories

A foundational concept in discussions of moral philosophy and ethics is that of the common morality [2], a term that refers to rules about right and wrong conduct that are widely accepted across cultures and moral traditions. Examples include prohibitions against lying, stealing, intentionally causing harm to others, keeping promises, respecting the rights of others. The common morality also values character traits that reflect adherence to desirable behavioral standards incorporated in rules of conduct. The idea of the common morality has been challenged, but for our purposes sets the stage for ethical theories and principles that can be applied to particular ethical problems. We will focus on three ethical theories that are most relevant to AI in healthcare (Table 12.1).

Table 12.1 Three ethical theories relevant to AI in healthcare

Ethical theory	Focus of the theory	Impact of use in AI	Challenges in use or deployment
Deontology	Adherence to moral rules and duties, emphasizing actions that are inherently right or wrong based on reasoning.	Ensures adherence to principles like transparency, informed consent, and privacy.	Need for clear ethical guidelines and policies that integrate deontological principles while allowing flexibility for innovation. May limit innovation if rules are too rigid.
Utilitarianism	Evaluates actions based on their outcomes, aiming to maximize overall happiness and minimize harm.	Maximizes the overall benefits of AI adoption, such as improved efficiency and healthcare access	Conduct thorough impact assessments to balance benefits and risks, ensuring that individual rights are not sacrificed for greater good. May overlook individual rights or unintended consequences.
Virtue ethics	Centers on the moral character and virtues of individuals, promoting ethical behavior based on traits like compassion, fairness, and integrity.	Encourages responsible development and use of AI, focusing on trust, compassion, and fairness	Need to provide training to cultivate ethical decision-making in developers and healthcare providers using AI. Lacks clear guidelines for practical implementation.

Utilitarianism

Utilitarianism derives from the work of nineteenth century English philosopher John Stuart Mill and others. The moral worth of actions is determined by their consequences or outcomes. If the benefits of the action exceed the harms the action is deemed appropriate and ethical. Public health policies often rely on this framework, for example, promoting vaccines which are known to have side effects and complications for small numbers of recipients while providing benefits to large numbers of people.

In the context of AI in healthcare, a utilitarian approach to an AI algorithm that analyzes patient data to identify those at risk for chronic diseases would support its deployment if it leads to improved health outcomes for a large number of patients, ultimately enhancing community health and reducing healthcare costs but if and only if these benefits exceed the risks or costs associated with their implementation. Thus, utilitarianism requires critical examination of both potential favorable and adverse consequences, such as over-reliance on AI to the detriment of the patient or the risk of biased outcomes that may adversely affect marginalized groups.

Deontology

Deontology, based on the work of Immanuel Kant, an eighteenth century German philosopher, focuses on adherence to moral duties and rules, positing that certain actions are inherently right or wrong regardless of their consequences. This ethical framework is particularly relevant when considering issues such as informed consent and patient autonomy in the deployment of AI technologies. For instance, when an AI system assists in diagnosing a patient's condition, healthcare providers have an ethical obligation to ensure that patients are fully informed about the AI's role in their care and the potential benefits and risks involved. A deontological approach would argue that even if the AI system significantly improves diagnostic accuracy (a potentially positive outcome), it is essential to respect the patient's right to make informed choices about their treatment. This obligation underscores the importance of transparency in AI applications and calls on healthcare professionals to prioritize ethical principles that uphold patient dignity and rights.

Virtue Ethics

Virtue ethics derives from the work of early Greek philosophers including Aristotle. It emphasizes the character and desirable moral qualities of individuals involved in decision-making, shifting focus away from rigid rules or consequences. In healthcare, this approach becomes particularly valuable as professionals navigate the complexities introduced by AI technologies. By cultivating virtues such as compassion, integrity, and fairness, healthcare professionals can facilitate ethical and patient-centered decision-making including with AI tools [3].

For example, a physician who uses an AI tool for treatment recommendations must not only consider the algorithm's output but also the ethical implications of those recommendations on the patient's overall well-being. A virtuous practitioner would approach the use of AI with a commitment to patient-centered care, ensuring that technology enhances the doctor-patient relationship and achieving patient goals as stated by the patient.

Principlism

Principlism or the four principles approach [2] derives from the ideas and theories described above. The four principles referenced by this term are:

Beneficence—a moral obligation to act to benefit others;
Non-maleficence—a moral obligation to avoid or prevent harm to others;
Respect for autonomy—an obligation to honor an individual's right to determine what is in their best interests;
Justice or Fairness—an obligation to ensure that benefits and burdens are distributed fairly and appropriately. Simply put, equals should be treated equally and unequals should be treated appropriately according to norms defined by a just society.

Broadening the Scope

Identifying and applying these major ethical frameworks to real-world scenarios can lead to better appreciation of the importance of ethical reasoning in the development and implementation of AI in healthcare and ensure that these technologies are utilized in ways that enhance patient care, uphold moral responsibilities, and promote equitable healthcare outcomes.

Ethical Concerns Associated with AI in Healthcare

The integration of AI in healthcare presents numerous opportunities for enhancing patient care and streamlining administrative processes. However, it also introduces a range of ethical concerns that healthcare professionals and other stakeholders must navigate. These often revolve around issues of consent, bias, accountability, accuracy, and the potential erosion of the patient-provider relationship. Understanding these challenges is critical for ensuring that AI technologies are implemented responsibly and ethically.

Patient- and Community-Centeredness

Patient-centered care, one of the six domains of healthcare quality established by the Institute of Medicine (now the National Academy of Medicine) means: "providing care that is respectful of and responsive to individual patient preferences, needs, and values and ensuring that patient values guide all clinical decisions." [4] This view is a keystone of contemporary views of the clinician-patient relationship and is best accomplished by a clinician whose values accord with this concept and acts accordingly, including when applying AI to decision-making.

Similarly, community-centered care requires consideration of the role of community values with respect to social determinants of health (SDOH) and other needs for purposes of policy-making and strategic planning when contemplating the adoption and implementation of AI tools in healthcare systems [5]. A large and growing body of knowledge has elucidated the impact of SDOH on the well-being of communities of disadvantaged populations. Significant differences in life span, rates of mortality, chronic and life-threatening conditions and many other health-related markers must be overcome, and AI will play a role in this.

Equity represents another domain of healthcare quality. The Agency for Healthcare Research and Quality (AHRQ) defines equity as "providing care that does not vary in quality because of personal characteristics such as gender, ethnicity, geographic location and socioeconomic status." [4] Biases, whether implicit or explicit, can be manifestations of inequity and adversely affect care [6]. AI systems are trained on massive amounts of data found throughout the internet, some of which may be inaccurate and reflect existing societal biases. An algorithm developed using data that does not fairly represent diverse populations may perpetuate or even exacerbate health disparities. To complicate matters, new evidence of heretofore unrealized bias is being found in AI algorithms with increasing frequency, and studies have shown that humans inherit AI biases [7], a dangerous finding. The ethical implications are profound, as healthcare providers must grapple with the responsibility of using tools that may unintentionally disadvantage certain patients or communities. Ensuring fairness and equity in AI-driven healthcare requires vigilance, ongoing re-evaluation, and the implementation of strategies to mitigate bias. It is not at all clear this can be fully overcome.

Informed consent is one of the primary ethical concerns in healthcare. As AI systems are increasingly used in diagnosis and treatment, patients must be made aware when these technologies influence their care. The vast amounts of data used to train algorithms may make it difficult for patients and even clinicians to understand the genesis of and rationale for AI recommendations. For instance, if an AI system suggests a particular treatment, the clinician is obligated to advise the patient of this and ensure that the patient understands the clinician's reasons for accepting or rejecting the recommendation. This dilemma raises questions about the adequacy of current consent processes, historically of concern, and whether patients can truly give informed consent when they or their healthcare providers may not fully understand the technology involved.

Privacy and security issues have risen to the forefront of ethical concerns because of the large amounts of personal health information (PHI) now held in electronic databases and being shared in clinical and research endeavors. Commercial interests developing AI tools draw on these large datasets, many of which, even when anonymized, present potential for accidental and criminal release or inappropriate use. There is at present very limited effective regulatory oversight, and with the extremely strong impulses in the market to develop AI rapidly, attention to security and privacy have not received the attention and constraint necessary to assure appropriate safeguards and prevent abuses [8].

Accuracy and Interpretability

Another concern is related to the accuracy or correctness of the information AI tools use and provide. It is now well-known that AI can fabricate data that appears authentic (hallucinations), use data that is wrong, or ignore data that should be considered, all of which can lead to flawed outputs with potential for harm. An active area of study and research, the sources of training data play a role in some of these deficiencies, but it is not yet known how to reliably identify such errors or prevent hallucinations. For this reason, the consensus is that AI is not ready for unsupervised use in most clinical settings.

A corollary to accuracy, interpretability represents the ease with which humans can understand and rely on the information and recommendations or decisions made by AI systems and is a sine qua non for trust and usability in the clinical setting [9]. Again, deficiencies in human understanding the workings of the "black box" of the algorithms contributes to this concern.

Accountability and Responsibility

As AI increasingly shapes the landscape of healthcare, questions of accountability and responsibility become paramount. There are numerous parties involved with AI in the clinical setting—healthcare providers, AI developers (individual and corporate), implementing institutions, and others. While the technologies promise to enhance efficiency, improve diagnostics, and personalize patient care, their use raises complex ethical and legal questions regarding who is accountable when AI systems fail or cause harm. Although autonomous AI systems where there is no human oversight are rare in healthcare, the technology is evolving rapidly, and these issues will become even more complex as the technology evolves. Establishing clear lines of accountability is essential to ensure patient safety and trust in these technologies.

For example, if an AI system incorrectly diagnoses a patient or suggests an inappropriate treatment, the clinician who relies on that AI must own responsibility for the ethical and legal ramifications of such a decision. The poor outcome may have resulted from, among a number of possibilities, poor quality of data by the model, inadequate training of the user, lack of understanding or transparency of the algorithm, or whether the end user adequately informed the patient about the AI's role in their care when deciding whether to proceed with the AI recommendation.

Developers of AI systems bear responsibility for ensuring that their technologies are safe, reliable, free from bias and used appropriately. This means conducting rigorous testing, maintaining transparency regarding how the algorithms work, and regularly updating systems to reflect new medical knowledge and practices and providing training and education for users. Healthcare organizations that implement AI technologies must also create an environment where ethical considerations are prioritized, ensuring that policies are in place to facilitate optimal use of the technology in the appropriate settings and to establish accountability procedures.

To enhance accountability and responsibility, several measures must be implemented. First, governments and regulators must establish clear regulatory frameworks defining the roles and responsibilities of stakeholders involved in AI development and deployment. These regulations should address issues such as data privacy, algorithmic transparency, and liability in cases of AI failure.

Second, education and training for clinicians and other users regarding the technical aspects of the models as well as ethical implications of their use must be provided. Practitioners must be equipped with the knowledge and skills necessary to critically assess AI recommendations, and this must coexist with a culture of informed decision-making that prioritizes patient welfare.

Finally, collaboration between AI developers, healthcare providers, patients, ethicists, business interests and regulatory bodies must be required to facilitate greater accountability. This can help ensure that AI technologies are developed and implemented with a clear focus on ethical considerations and patient safety.

Erosion of Trust and the Clinician Patient Relationship

The potential for erosion of the patient-provider relationship poses an ethical concern as AI becomes more integrated into healthcare. The human connection between patients and providers is foundational to effective care and is built on trust and empathy. As AI technologies take on more roles in diagnosis and treatment, there is a risk that the personal aspect of healthcare may diminish. Patients may feel they are interacting more with machines than with human caregivers, potentially impacting their willingness to engage in open communication about their health. Healthcare professionals must find ways to balance the efficiency and accuracy of AI with the need for compassionate, personalized care that recognizes the emotional and psychological aspects of health.

Another aspect of this issue is the effect of AI on the skills and education of clinicians. It is already known that the exponential increase in medical knowledge poses challenges for keeping up with new information [10]. While AI will support many clinical processes—diagnosis, recommending treatment plans, performing robotic surgery, etc—it is crucial to evaluate whether reliance on these technologies may inadvertently lead to complacency among healthcare professionals, potentially undermining their cognitive and procedural skills, clinical judgment and expertise.

Evaluate AI's Impact on Patient Care

It is now clear that these technologies must fulfill their promise while adhering to rigorous ethical standards. Only then can the benefits truly outweigh the challenges associated with AI, including its effects on patient outcomes, healthcare accessibility, and the patient-provider relationship.

With regard to diagnosis, AI algorithms can analyze vast amounts of data and identify patterns that may be difficult for human clinicians to detect. At present, the most successful uses of AI in diagnosis have been in assessing visual images, i.e., radiologic, ophthalmologic, dermatologic. For instance, AI applications in radiology can assist in identifying anomalies in imaging studies, such as tumors or fractures, with a high degree of accuracy. AI systems can match or even surpass the diagnostic performance of radiologists in certain contexts, leading to earlier detection of conditions and potentially improved outcomes for patients. However, AI interpretations of images is not yet at a level of accuracy and reliability to dispense with human clinician oversight. In addition, diagnosis in the cognitive realm is not nearly as highly evolved although development is moving rapidly [11].

Besides enhancing diagnosis, AI can personalize treatment plans by using individual patient data from traditional sources like medical records, including genetic information, lifestyle factors, medical history; it can also incorporate data from newer personal health monitoring devices, the sophistication and use of which is growing rapidly. This personalized approach allows tailoring of interventions to meet patients' specific needs and more effective treatment outcomes. With the ability to quickly and effectively compare an index patient's symptoms and signs may help to arrive at a diagnosis more quickly.

AI also has the potential to improve healthcare accessibility, particularly in underserved populations. Many patients are comfortable using the internet to look for information related to symptoms and diseases, and as AI chatbots and virtual assistants become more familiar and reliable, their use to obtain medical advice, navigate health concerns and find appropriate resources will grow. Telemedicine platforms as well as personal health monitoring devices powered by AI will facilitate remote consultations, allowing patients in rural or remote areas to access specialist care that might otherwise be unavailable. It is essential that these technologies be proven to enhance access, not create new barriers, particularly for individuals who may lack the technological literacy or resources to utilize AI-driven platforms effectively.

Monitoring AI in Healthcare

Monitoring AI systems is essential for ensuring their ongoing effectiveness and safety. Continuous oversight can be achieved through several strategies, including regular audits of AI algorithms and transformers, monitoring for discrepancies between AI recommendations and actual patient outcomes, and employing human oversight in decision-making processes. Establishing clear performance metrics is crucial, allowing healthcare providers to assess the reliability and accuracy of AI recommendations over time.

Additionally, transparency in AI operations is vital. Developers should provide clear documentation regarding the data and methodologies used to train AI systems, as well as how those systems arrive at their conclusions. This information should be accessible to healthcare professionals, enabling them to understand the reasoning behind AI-generated recommendations and facilitating informed discussions with patients. Implementing feedback loops that allow healthcare professionals to report adverse outcomes or concerns about AI systems are essential to further enhance monitoring efforts.

Guidelines to Effect Ethically Responsible Use of AI

As AI technologies have advanced, various organizations and regulatory bodies have proposed guidelines aimed at ensuring responsible use in healthcare; notable examples include:

- The World Health Organization (WHO), in 2021, released a draft report outlining principles for the ethical use of AI in health [12]. Citing 6 core principles, this document emphasizes fairness, transparency, and accountability, urging stakeholders to prioritize ethical considerations throughout the development and implementation of AI systems [13].
- The U.S. Food and Drug Administration (FDA) has established frameworks for regulating AI and machine learning software as medical devices [14, 15]. This framework includes premarket assessment, post-market surveillance, and a focus on ensuring that AI systems provide accurate and reliable results.
- The European Union's General Data Protection Regulation (GDPR), while not exclusively focused on AI, establishes principles for data protection and privacy that significantly impact the use of AI in healthcare, particularly in terms of informed consent, data minimization, and individual rights [16].

Despite these initiatives, there remains a lack of comprehensive, standardized ethics guidelines specifically tailored to the unique challenges posed by AI in healthcare. To address these gaps, it is necessary to establish a set of ethical guidelines that encapsulate the complexities of AI applications in this field.

Proposed Ethical Guidelines for AI in Healthcare

The ethical guidelines for AI in healthcare should include the following key principles:

- Transparency: AI algorithms should be transparent, allowing healthcare providers and patients to understand how its recommendations and decisions are made. This includes clear documentation of the data used, the rationale behind AI recommendations, and the limitations of the technology.
- Accountability: Stakeholders, including healthcare providers, AI developers, and organizations, must be held responsible and accountable for the outcomes of AI systems.
- Fairness and Equity: AI systems must be designed to minimize bias and ensure equitable access to care for all populations. This requires using diverse training data that accurately reflects the demographics of the patient populations and mechanisms to monitor and address disparities in AI outcomes.
- Informed Consent: Patients should be fully informed about the use of AI in their care, including potential risks, benefits, and how their data will be used. Informed consent processes must be clear and understandable, empowering patients to make informed decisions.
- Data Privacy and Security: Robust measures must be implemented to protect patient data and ensure compliance with relevant privacy regulations. This includes secure data storage, anonymization techniques, and strict access controls.
- Continuous Monitoring and Improvement: AI systems should be subject to ongoing evaluation and monitoring to ensure they remain effective and ethically sound over time. This includes regular audits of algorithm performance, safety assessments, and updates to reflect the latest medical knowledge.

Implementation of Ethical Guidelines

Implementing ethical guidelines for AI in healthcare requires a multifaceted approach:

- Stakeholder Engagement: Engaging a wide range of stakeholders, including patients, healthcare providers, AI developers, ethicists, regulators and policymakers, is crucial for developing guidelines that address diverse perspectives and needs.

- Training and Education: Healthcare professionals should receive training on the ethical implications of AI technologies. This education should encompass not only technical understanding but also the moral and social responsibilities associated with AI use in patient care, research and education.
- Institutional Policies: Healthcare organizations should develop internal policies that align with ethical guidelines, incorporating them into their governance structures and operational practices. This includes establishing ethics committees to review AI projects and decisions.
- Regulatory Frameworks: Governments and regulatory bodies should create comprehensive legal frameworks that support the implementation of ethical guidelines. This includes setting standards for AI technologies, monitoring compliance, and enforcing accountability mechanisms.

Monitoring Ethical Guidelines

Effective monitoring of ethical guidelines is essential for ensuring adherence and addressing emerging issues:

- Independent Oversight Bodies: Establishing independent organizations or committees to oversee AI implementations in healthcare can enhance accountability. These bodies should be tasked with reviewing compliance, conducting audits, and addressing ethical concerns and given appropriate authority to be effective.
- Feedback Mechanisms: Creating channels for healthcare providers and patients to report concerns about AI systems fosters transparency and accountability. These mechanisms should allow stakeholders to provide input on AI performance, effectiveness, and ethical considerations.
- Public Reporting: Regularly publishing reports on AI outcomes, biases, and ethical considerations can promote transparency and build public trust. These reports should include metrics on how AI systems impact patient care and any actions taken to address ethical concerns.

Evaluating Ethical Guidelines

Evaluating the effectiveness of ethical guidelines for AI in healthcare is crucial for continuous improvement:

- Performance Metrics: Establishing clear metrics for evaluating AI systems can help determine their effectiveness and ethical compliance. These metrics should assess outcomes related to patient safety, treatment efficacy, equity, and transparency.

- Patient and Provider Surveys: Conducting regular surveys of patients and healthcare providers can provide insights into their experiences with AI technologies, including perceived benefits, concerns, and areas for improvement.
- Longitudinal Studies: Long-term studies can help assess the impact of AI on patient care over time, identifying trends, benefits, and potential ethical issues that arise with continued use.

Impact of Ethical Guidelines

The implementation of robust ethical guidelines for AI in healthcare should yield significant positive outcomes:

- Improved Patient Safety: By ensuring that AI systems are transparent, accountable, and continuously monitored, the risk of adverse events and misdiagnoses can be reduced, ultimately improving patient safety.
- Increased Trust: When patients and providers understand the ethical framework guiding AI technologies, it can foster trust in these systems. This trust is essential for encouraging the adoption of AI tools in clinical practice.
- Equitable Care: Guidelines that prioritize fairness and equity can help address health disparities, ensuring that all populations benefit from advancements in AI technology.
- Enhanced Innovation: A clear ethical framework can stimulate responsible innovation in AI development, encouraging researchers and developers to create technologies that prioritize patient welfare and adhere to ethical standards.
- Informed Decision-Making: With an emphasis on informed consent and transparency, patients can make better-informed decisions about their care, leading to improved patient engagement and satisfaction.

In conclusion, the establishment of ethical guidelines for AI in healthcare is essential for ensuring responsible use of these technologies. By addressing current policies, proposing key principles, implementing robust strategies, and evaluating their impact, stakeholders can work together to navigate the complexities of AI while prioritizing patient safety, equity, and trust. As AI continues to evolve, ongoing dialogue and collaboration among healthcare professionals, technologists, ethicists, and patients will be crucial for adapting these guidelines to meet emerging challenges and opportunities in the field.

Outlook and Conclusions

This chapter on Ethical Theories for AI in Healthcare provides a comprehensive exploration of the fundamental ethical principles that guide the integration of artificial intelligence into the healthcare landscape. As AI technologies become increasingly prevalent in diagnostic tools, treatment recommendations, and patient management, understanding the ethical implications of their use is essential for ensuring responsible practices and safeguarding patient welfare.

The chapter begins by outlining key ethical theories relevant to AI in healthcare, including utilitarianism, deontology, and virtue ethics. Utilitarianism emphasizes the consequences of actions, advocating for decisions that maximize overall happiness or benefit. In the context of AI, this theory suggests that AI applications should be evaluated based on their potential to improve patient outcomes and public health. For instance, a predictive algorithm that accurately identifies high-risk patients for preventive care could be justified from a utilitarian perspective, as it enhances overall health benefits.

In contrast, deontology focuses on the morality of actions themselves rather than their outcomes. This theory posits that certain ethical principles must be upheld, regardless of the consequences. In the realm of AI, deontological considerations may include the obligation to obtain informed consent from patients before utilizing AI technologies, ensuring transparency in how AI systems operate, and maintaining patient privacy and autonomy. By adhering to these principles, healthcare providers can fulfill their ethical obligations to patients, whether or not AI systems offer efficiency or improved outcomes.

The chapter also explores virtue ethics, which emphasizes the importance of character and the moral virtues of healthcare professionals across many disciplines in their interactions with AI technologies. This perspective encourages practitioners to cultivate qualities such as empathy, integrity, and responsibility when using AI in patient care. For example, a physician who approaches AI recommendations with a critical mindset, questioning their validity and considering the individual needs of patients, exemplifies the virtue of prudence. By fostering a virtuous approach, healthcare professionals can ensure that the integration of AI aligns with the core values of the medical profession and meets patient needs.

Moreover, the chapter addresses ethical dilemmas arising from AI applications in healthcare, such as those related to bias, accountability, and the patient-provider relationship. Bias in AI algorithms can lead to disparities in care, highlighting the need for equitable AI systems that serve diverse populations. The chapter emphasizes the importance of ongoing monitoring and evaluation of AI technologies to identify and mitigate biases, ensuring that all patients receive fair treatment.

Accountability is another critical issue discussed in the chapter. The responsibility for AI-driven decisions must be clearly defined, encompassing healthcare providers, AI developers, and organizations. Establishing accountability mechanisms is essential for addressing ethical concerns and fostering trust in AI technologies among patients and practitioners alike.

The chapter concludes by stressing the significance of ethical frameworks in guiding the development and implementation of AI in healthcare. By incorporating ethical theories into practice, healthcare professionals can navigate the complexities of AI, ensuring that patient welfare remains at the forefront of technological advancements. The chapter ultimately advocates for a collaborative approach that engages stakeholders across the entire spectrum of healthcare—including patients, clinicians, ethicists, technologists, administrators, regulators, policy makers and the public at large—in the ongoing discourse surrounding the ethical use of AI in healthcare.

In summary, the chapter on Ethical Theories for AI in Healthcare provides a thorough examination of the ethical frameworks that inform the integration of AI into medical practice. By exploring utilitarianism, deontology, and virtue ethics, the chapter equips healthcare professionals with the necessary tools to make informed decisions in an increasingly complex landscape, ensuring that AI serves as a force for good patient care.

A final caveat: The field of AI in healthcare is evolving at breakneck speed. While ethics evolves more slowly than the technology, constant vigilance and life-long learning will be required to maintain an ethical response to the new challenges that come along. Some of these challenges will be dramatic and paradigm shifting, forcing considerations of existential questions for humanity.

Useful Resources

Stanford Encyclopedia of Ethics: Ethics of Artificial Intelligence and Robotics—https://plato.stanford.edu/entries/ethics-ai/.

NEJM AI Grand Rounds podcast—https://ai-podcast.nejm.org: informal conversations with a variety of unique experts exploring the deep issues at the intersection of artificial intelligence, machine learning, and medicine.

JAMA+ AI (Journal of the American Medical Association AI podcast)—https://jamanetwork.com/channels/ai: Resources for "advances in the application of artificial intelligence in medicine—from clinical practice to research to education.

The Road to Accountable AI with Kevin Weerbach—https://podcasts.apple.com/us/podcast/the-road-to-accountable-ai/id1739948118: Explores the intersection of technology, law and ethics with Professor Werback of the Wharton School and his guests.

Matheny M, Thadaney Israni S, Ahmed M, Whicher D, editors. Artificial intelligence in health care: the hope, the hype, the promise, the peril. Washington, DC: National Academy of Medicine; 2022.

Review Questions

1. Describe the three major ethical theories discussed in the chapter. Compare and contrast how each theory would approach the ethical challenges posed by AI in healthcare. Provide an example for each.
2. Application of Ethical Principles: How can utilitarianism be applied to assess the effectiveness of an AI-driven diagnostic tool? Provide an example that illustrates this application.
3. Deontological Considerations: According to deontological ethics, what obligations do healthcare providers have when implementing AI technologies? Discuss how these obligations might affect patient consent processes.
4. Virtue Ethics in Practice: How does virtue ethics inform the behavior of healthcare professionals when using AI? Provide an example of a virtuous action that a healthcare provider might take in the context of AI-assisted patient care.

5. Ethical Dilemmas and Solutions: What are some of the ethical dilemmas associated with AI in healthcare that the chapter highlights? Discuss potential solutions or strategies to address these dilemmas while ensuring patient safety and equity.

Answers to Review Questions

1. The three major ethical theories commonly discussed are deontology, utilitarianism, and virtue ethics. Each offers a distinct perspective on addressing the ethical challenges posed by AI in healthcare:

   (a) *Deontology:*

   - Approach: Deontology focuses on adherence to moral rules and duties. In the context of AI, it emphasizes respecting patient autonomy, privacy, and informed consent. Even if an AI system significantly improves outcomes, it must align with ethical principles that prioritize patient rights and transparency.
   - Example: A deontological approach would argue that patients must have the right to understand and consent to how AI influences their care, regardless of its efficiency.

   (b) *Utilitarianism:*

   - Approach: Utilitarianism evaluates actions based on their outcomes, aiming to maximize overall benefits and minimize harm. With AI in healthcare, this theory supports implementing systems that enhance diagnostic accuracy and treatment efficiency, provided the overall good outweighs potential risks.
   - Example: A utilitarian perspective might justify the widespread use of AI if it reduces medical errors and improves population health, even if some individual risks or ethical concerns arise.

   (c) *Virtue Ethics:*

   - Approach: Virtue ethics centers on the moral character of individuals and actions that reflect virtues like compassion, fairness, and integrity. In healthcare AI, this approach encourages developers and providers to act with integrity, prioritizing patient well-being over profit or efficiency.
   - Example: Virtue ethics would focus on whether the use of AI promotes trust, empathy, and fairness in patient care rather than solely emphasizing outcomes or rules.

   (d) *Comparison:*

   - Deontology vs. Utilitarianism: Deontology emphasizes strict adherence to rules and rights, while utilitarianism prioritizes outcomes, even if some rules are compromised.
   - Virtue Ethics vs. Others: Virtue ethics focuses on the character and intentions behind decisions, contrasting with the rule-based deontology and outcome-driven utilitarianism.

Together, these theories provide a comprehensive framework for navigating the ethical complexities of AI in healthcare, balancing principles, outcomes, and moral character.

2. *Application of Utilitarianism to AI-Driven Diagnostic Tools*

   Utilitarianism evaluates actions based on their consequences, aiming to maximize overall benefits while minimizing harm. When applied to assess the effectiveness of an AI-driven diagnostic tool, utilitarianism focuses on the tool's ability to improve patient outcomes, reduce diagnostic errors, and enhance healthcare efficiency for the greatest number of people.

   Example:

   Consider an AI system designed to detect early-stage lung cancer from radiological images. A utilitarian assessment would involve evaluating the tool's net impact on patient health and healthcare systems:

   (a) Benefits:

      - The AI tool increases diagnostic accuracy, identifying 95% of early-stage cases compared to 80% by human radiologists. This leads to earlier treatment and higher survival rates.
      - It reduces diagnostic time, allowing radiologists to focus on complex cases, thereby improving overall efficiency.
      - Widespread adoption could lower healthcare costs by minimizing advanced-stage treatments.

   (b) Potential Harms:

      - The tool has a 5% false-positive rate, potentially leading to unnecessary anxiety and additional testing for some patients.
      - Over-reliance on AI might reduce opportunities for radiologists to refine their diagnostic skills.

   (c) Weighing Outcomes:

      A utilitarian analysis concludes that the tool's significant improvements in survival rates and healthcare efficiency outweigh the manageable risks of false positives and skill erosion, justifying its adoption.

      Conclusion:

      Through utilitarianism, the effectiveness of an AI diagnostic tool is assessed by balancing its benefits and harms across the broader population. This approach ensures that decisions prioritize maximizing positive outcomes for patients and healthcare systems as a whole.

3. Deontological Considerations and Obligations in Implementing AI Technologies

   According to deontological ethics, healthcare providers are obligated to adhere to moral principles and duties regardless of the outcomes. When implementing AI technologies, these obligations include:

   (a) Respecting Patient Autonomy: Providers must ensure patients have the right to make informed decisions about their care. This requires transparency about how AI technologies are used and their potential benefits and risks.

(b) Ensuring Fairness and Equity: Providers must ensure that AI tools are applied without bias and that all patients receive equitable treatment, regardless of socioeconomic status, ethnicity, or other factors.
(c) Maintaining Confidentiality: Providers must safeguard patient data used by AI systems, ensuring compliance with privacy regulations and protecting sensitive information from misuse.

Impact on Patient Consent Processes:

Deontological ethics necessitates that patient consent processes be robust and transparent when incorporating AI technologies. This could involve:

- Providing Clear Explanations: Patients must be informed about the role of AI in their diagnosis or treatment, including how the technology works, its limitations, and potential risks.
- Offering Alternatives: Patients should have the choice to opt out of AI-driven care if they prefer traditional methods, ensuring their autonomy is respected.
- Documenting Consent Thoroughly: Consent must be explicitly obtained and documented, particularly when AI involves data sharing or automated decision-making.

By prioritizing these obligations, healthcare providers can uphold ethical principles, fostering trust and ensuring that AI technologies are implemented in a manner that respects patient rights and dignity.

4. Virtue Ethics in Practice: Guiding Healthcare Professionals in AI-Assisted Care

Virtue ethics focuses on the character and moral virtues of individuals, guiding them to act in ways that reflect qualities like compassion, integrity, and fairness. When healthcare professionals use AI, virtue ethics informs their behavior by encouraging actions that prioritize the well-being and dignity of patients over convenience, profit, or uncritical reliance on technology.

Example of a Virtuous Action:

A healthcare provider is using an AI diagnostic tool to interpret a patient's radiology scans. The AI suggests a high probability of a serious condition, but the provider notices inconsistencies in the broader clinical picture. Instead of blindly accepting the AI's recommendation, the provider takes the time to:

- Verify the Results: Conduct additional tests or seek a second opinion to confirm the diagnosis, demonstrating diligence and prudence.
- Communicate with Empathy: Explain the situation to the patient in clear, compassionate terms, acknowledging the limitations of AI while reassuring the patient of their commitment to providing the best care.
- Act with Integrity: Balance reliance on AI with their professional judgment, ensuring decisions reflect both technological insights and human expertise.

By embodying virtues like prudence, empathy, and integrity, the healthcare provider ensures that AI is used as a tool to enhance, not replace, human-centered care, ultimately fostering trust and ethical decision-making in patient care.

5. Ethical Dilemmas and Solutions in AI Healthcare

   The chapter highlights several ethical dilemmas associated with AI in healthcare, including:

   (a) Bias and Inequity: AI systems may inherit biases from the data they are trained on, leading to unequal treatment or misdiagnoses for certain patient groups.

      - Solution: Implement rigorous bias audits during the development and deployment of AI tools. Use diverse and representative datasets, and involve multidisciplinary teams, including ethicists, to ensure fairness and equity.

   (b) Lack of Transparency: Many AI systems function as "black boxes," making it difficult for healthcare providers to understand how decisions are made.

      - Solution: Advocate for explainable AI (XAI) systems that provide clear, interpretable insights into their decision-making processes. Transparency ensures that providers and patients can trust AI-driven recommendations.

   (c) Accountability: Determining who is responsible when an AI system causes harm is often unclear.

      - Solution: Establish clear accountability frameworks that assign responsibilities to AI developers, healthcare providers, and institutions. These frameworks should be codified in legal and organizational policies.

   (d) Patient Privacy and Data Security: AI systems require access to large amounts of sensitive patient data, increasing the risk of breaches and misuse.

      - Solution: Use advanced encryption methods, anonymization techniques, and strict access controls to protect patient data. Compliance with data privacy laws like HIPAA or GDPR is essential.

   (e) Scope Creep and Over-Reliance: Healthcare providers might over-rely on AI systems, potentially neglecting their own clinical judgment.

      - Solution: Emphasize training and education for healthcare professionals on AI's capabilities and limitations. Encourage AI to be viewed as a supportive tool rather than a replacement for human expertise.

Ensuring Patient Safety and Equity:

By integrating these strategies, healthcare organizations can mitigate the ethical risks of AI while fostering trust, improving patient outcomes, and ensuring that technology serves the broader goal of equitable and safe care. A proactive approach involving continuous monitoring, stakeholder collaboration, and adherence to ethical principles is critical for navigating these challenges effectively.

Appendix: Four-Box Approach to Analyzing Ethics Cases in AI

We offer here an approach for performing an ethical analysis when confronting an ethics concern in AI. It takes into consideration the four ethics principles of Beauchamp and Childress, namely beneficence, non-maleficense, autonomy and justice/equity, and also the six core principles enunciated in the WHO statement, namely autonomy; promotion of human well-being, human safety, and the public interest; transparency, explainability, and intelligibility; responsibility and accountability; inclusiveness and equity; and promotion of AI that is responsive and sustainable.

Be aware that this is a suggested approach. It has not been rigorously vetted in practice.

A four-box approach to analyzing ethics cases in AI	
Technical Indications: **The Principles of Beneficence and Non-maleficence** 1. What is the AI ethics issue?[a] 2. What are the goals of the AI tool/algorithm? 3. What are the alternative approaches to accomplish the goal? 4. What are the probabilities of success of the various approaches? 5. Which option has the least likelihood of adverse consequences or harm? 6. In sum, how can this tool/algorithm benefit patients or processes and how can harm be avoided?	**Preferences of Patient or Other Beneficiary (POB) of use of the TOOL The Principle of Respect for Autonomy** 1. Has the POB been informed of or is aware of the benefits, risks and alternatives to the tool. 2. Does the POB have decisional capacity to understand the benefits, risks and alternatives? 3. What is the preferred option of the POB or other decision-maker?[b] 4. Is there any valid reason to override the decision-makers choice?
Quality of Outcomes: The Principles of Beneficence, Nonmaleficence, and Respect for Autonomy 1. What are the prospects for a successful outcome with and without the tool/algorithm and what is the worst case for either option ***from the end-user's or patient's perspective***? 2. Are there biases—conscious, unconscious or unknown as well as differential power relationships between or among the interested parties and decision-maker(s)—that could prejudice any of the parties? Consider a third party or ethics consultation. 3. What ethical issues arise concerning improving or enhancing the end-user's outcome? 4. What kinds of quality-of-outcome assessments raise questions regarding favoring or rejecting a choice?	**Contextual Features: The Principles of Justice and Fairness** 1. Are there professional, inter-professional or business interests that might create conflicts of interest in the design or choice of tool/algorithm? 2. What is the most cost-effective option to achieve the goal? 3. What is the most cost-effective option to achieve the goal? 4. Are there parties other than clinicians and patients who have a stake in the outcome? If so, how will those interests be prioritized justly. 5. What are the limits imposed by legitimate interests of third parties? 6. Are there financial factors that create conflicts of interest? 7. Are there problems of allocation of scarce health resources that might affect the decisions? 8. Are there legal, regulatory, research, educational, public health, safety or other factors that should be considered?

Adapted from Jonsen et al. [17], https://depts.washington.edu/bhdept/ethics-medicine/bioethics-tools

[a]Refers to the reason(s) an ethics consultation regarding the AI tool is being sought

[b]Refers to the option preferred by the end user for whom the ethics question is being considered. It could mean whether to use AI at all or to use it to supplement and/or complement clinician's or developer's decision or to weigh in when there are multiple options being considered, as a tie breaker, for example, by providing information to assist in the choice. Of course, the final end user—patient or clinician or developer, for example—would have the final say

References

1. Chen JH. Who's training whom? A physician's surprising encounter with ChatGPT. Stanford Medicine. 10 Nov 2023. https://stanmed.stanford.edu/surprising-chatgpt-revelation/. Accessed 23 Jan 2025.
2. Beauchamp TL, Childress JF. Principles of biomedical ethics. 8th ed. New York: Oxford University Press; 2019.
3. Victor A. Medium: Aristotle's virtue ethics as a blueprint for AI governance. 4 Jan 2025. https://adammvictor.com/aristotle/aristotle-virtue-ethics-ai-governance/. Accessed 9 Jan 2025.
4. Institute of Medicine (IOM). Crossing the quality chasm: a new health system for the 21st century. Washington, DC: National Academy Press; 2001. Accessed via https://www.ahrq.gov/talkingquality/measures/six-domains.html.
5. National Academies of Sciences, Engineering, and Medicine. The current state of racial and ethnic disparities in health care. In: Nass SJ, Amankwah FK, DeVoe JE, et al., editors. Ending unequal treatment: strategies to achieve equitable health care and optimal health for all. Washington, DC: National Academies Press (US); 2024 Aug 23.
6. Min A. Artificial intelligence and bias: challenges, implications and remedies. J Soc Res. 2023;2:3808–17.
7. Vicente L, Matute H. Humans inherit artificial intelligence biases. Sci Rep. 2023;13:15737. https://doi.org/10.1038/s41598-023-42384-8.
8. US Presidential Executive Order 14110 of October 30, 2023. Safe, secure, and trustworthy development and use of artificial intelligence – rescinded as of 01/20/2025.
9. Ennab M, Mcheick H. Enhancing interpretability and accuracy of AI models in healthcare: a comprehensive review on challenges and future directions. Front Robot AI. 2024;11:1444763. https://www.frontiersin.org/journals/robotics-and-ai/articles/10.3389/frobt.2024.1444763.
10. Densen P. Challenges and opportunities facing medical education. Trans Am Clin Climatol Assoc. 2011;122:48–58. PMID: 21686208; PMCID: PMC3116346.
11. CoDEx Strategic Plan. https://codex.ucsf.edu/news/announcing-ucsf-codex-strategic-plan. Accessed 22 Jan 2025.
12. WHO. Ethics and governance of artificial intelligence for health: WHO guidance. Geneva: World Health Organization; 2021. License: CC BY-NC-SA 3.0 IGO.
13. WHO 6 core principles for ethics in healthcare: (1) protect autonomy; (2) promote human well-being, human safety, and the public interest; (3) ensure transparency, explainability, and intelligibility; (4) foster responsibility and accountability; (5) ensure inclusiveness and equity; (6) promote AI that is responsive and sustainable.
14. Warraich HJ, Tazbaz T, Califf RM. FDA perspective on the regulation of artificial intelligence in health care and biomedicine. JAMA. 2025;333(3):241–7.
15. NSF. FDA draft guidance on use of AI to support regulatory decision-making for drug and biological products. 20 Jan 2025. https://www.nsf.org/life-science-news/fda-draft-guidance-on-use-of-ai-to-support-regulatory-decision-making-for-drug-and-biological-products. Accessed 22 Jan 2025.
16. General Data Protection Regulation. https://gdpr-info.eu.
17. Jonsen AR, Siegler M, Winslade W. Clinical ethics. 7th ed. McGraw-Hill; 2010.

Part V
Conclusions and Outlook

Chapter 13
Artificial and Human Intelligence: Data as Bridge Builders

Ursula H. Hübner, Giovanni Rubeis, and Marion J. Ball

Learning Objectives

- To understand the pivotal role of data for AI and bridging artificial and human intelligence
- To understand the specific nature of medical and health data
- To understand the meaning of FAIR data
- To understand data quality and how to measure it
- To understand health data governance and data stewards

Key Terms

- Small data sets
- Data quality
- FAIR data
- OMOP Common Data Model
- Data governance
- Data steward

Summary

Data in their dual role as the representatives of the real world and as fuel for AI applications constitute the bridge between the two worlds of artificial intelligence and human intelligence. Data in medicine and healthcare are characterized by many peculiarities, such as limited access due to privacy and security demands, scarcity in

U. H. Hübner (✉)
School of Business Management and Social Sciences, Osnabrück University of Applied Sciences, Osnabrück, Germany

G. Rubeis
Institute of Ethics and History of Medicine, University of Greifswald, Greifswald, Germany

M. J. Ball
Center for Innovation in Health Informatics (CIHI), University of Texas at Arlington, Arlington, TX, USA

U. H. Hübner et al. (eds.), *Bridging Artificial and Human Intelligence*, Health Informatics, https://doi.org/10.1007/978-3-032-11938-4_13

case of rare diseases, but also by the lack of interoperability. The FAIR principles and standardization effort, such as the OMOP Common Data Model, offer solutions to manage data so that they can be used for AI developments. As data quality is key, health data governance policies have to be put into place. The future of robust and reliable AI in healthcare is coupled with dataware, the availability of very large health data spaces.

Data: A Short Summary of the Previous Chapters

Although artificial and human intelligence share the conceptual idea of intelligence, they represent different types of realms with their own tools and procedures. While AI dwells on huge amounts of data, humans are specialized to make the most out of a scarcity of data. Humans are good at seeing the big picture, while machines analyze the details. These realms need bridges to coexist as well as to reach out to each other in a meaningful manner, support each other, and contribute to the advancement of healthcare. For these bridges to become sustainable, they need to be built by all of the relevant stakeholders in the healthcare ecosystem, not only by AI specialists. In this chapter, we argue that data are the bricks for the bridges that are meant to align artificial and human intelligence. Data serve as representatives of the human shaped physical world. Data are also the essence of training AI models. By analogy with hardware, software and peopleware, we speak about dataware as the fourth pillar of digitalization. This argumentation is supported by the different viewpoints of the chapters in this book as summarized in the following.

AI's long scientific history, which started with human heuristics and knowledge implanted explicitly into digital systems, is more and more converging toward applying data-driven methods. As machine learning and deep learning become the prevailing paradigm of AI, learning through algorithms and data has become the agency of acting intelligently. In the augmentation scenario—as opposed to the automation scenario—humans and machines interact in the data universe: Humans are producing and procuring real world data according to standards and principles. They are labeling data for supervised AI methods, assessing the limitations and biases of datasets, and finally checking them. These activities all happen when humans are acting in their role as consumers or users, professionals driving AI (translators), and developers of AI. These activities also reverberate in educational recommendations where different types of AI competencies correspond with these roles. When humans take care of data this does not necessarily mean that they abandon their inherent way of perceiving the world, processing information, and solving problems.

The term "datafication", which is often used as a portentous sign of losing the human touch of caring, denotes merely a process of describing an entity through data. Beyond inspecting the world through the data lens, humans may still be emotional and empathetic when treating patients and trying to maintain a good patient-provider relationship. Bringing social and emotional intelligence to the table does not preclude being precise, fact-oriented, and meticulous when it comes to data. These two sides of the same coin are often misconceived.

Another misunderstanding is that technology, including AI, does not concern the higher echelons of an organization. The same could be said about data that bring about innovation. Data are not simply technical details but rather the asset of an organization. Upon this new gold, medical and nursing knowledge can be developed. This type of asset management is an integral part and an obligation of the new leadership. Similarly, leadership commitment to any disruptive change such as AI belongs to the core determinants for the successful outcomes of an AI implementation. When AI tools are bought, a thorough understanding of the data and their quality underlying the model applied is essential to appraise the limitations and benefits of the tool. Sometimes your own organizational data must be incorporated when customizing an AI tool, e.g., a chatbot. Conversely, when models are developed instead of being bought, providing high quality data is the key determinant on the path to the success of the AI application—be it in medicine, nursing, gerontology, or in workflow management as seen in the case studies of this book. The more relevant data about a patient that are known, the higher the chance is to provide personalized medicine and tailored care offers.

In a Learning Health System, data typically reside in electronic health records or registries that need to be interoperable when data are shared across systems, departments, institutions, and countries. Interoperability embraces technical aspects, such as protocols, but also semantic aspects, such as using the same terminology or coding system, and also those aspects of data models that describe the properties, structure, and interrelationships of the data. Interoperability is a concerted effort of standardization bodies, politics, vendors, healthcare institutions, and users. In the era of AI, interoperability and accessibility of data in healthcare is more necessary than ever before.

Although data are praised as the new gold, they intricately may possess features described as biases. These biases in data sets not only cause invalid AI models but they can also exacerbate health disparities. Biases surrounding data may result from incorrect, inconsistent, and irrelevant data, likewise from variables that are meaningless in this context or simply missing. In case of supervised learning, data need to be labeled, which can require human experts to annotate the data. This is a process that is not only cumbersome but also error prone. While debiasing strategies comprise technical measures, they also call for AI evaluation to reveal the output, outcome, and impact on patient care, the organization, and society. As data are produced in a certain context, data must be accompanied by metadata describing their provenance and formation.

The nature of the data in a domain can only be evaluated by domain experts. Therefore, healthcare professionals of various specialties and professional backgrounds are obliged to evolve from passive consumers to active participants. Liability for diagnostic, treatment, and care decisions is another reason that puts healthcare professionals in the "driver's seat" rather than leaving them in the "passenger's seat". Furthermore, patients are concerned about playing an active role. When non-anonymized data are to be processed, informed consent is required by law in many countries—in case there is no legal base for the processing. Other data protection issues and measures are similarly covered by law, restricting the unfettered use of sensitive personal data. The degree to which these measures are stipulated ranges from very strict to rather flexible. The pertaining laws directly impact the opportunities to use data for model training.

As humans, lawmakers are the critical gatekeepers who define the conditions under which data processing is possible and AI applications are conformant with the regulations. In a greater sense, laws also reflect the ethical concerns about the loss of privacy, security, autonomy, and other risks. However, not all ethical issues could be materialized in laws. Therefore, they should be embedded in ethical guidelines for AI. They are the basis for evaluating and monitoring AI developments according to principles of data and output transparency, stakeholder accountability, fairness, and equity due to a minimization of biases—among others.

The legal and ethical perspectives on data for AI highlight the potential power that humans have to shape the way artificial intelligence is used to advance healthcare and improve the patient-provider relationship. Having said that, the breakneck speed of new developments in AI often exceeds the time needed for ethical discourses to take place in society and laws to be put in place. Health professionals must develop their own pattern of judgments. Knowledge about the role of high-quality data and oversight about the pipeline from data capture to data processing empower health professionals to critically appraise the output of AI applications.

The Nature of Medical and Health Data

The golden rule of "the more data there are, the better the models will be" for developing AI models has been demonstrated well outside of healthcare—as exemplified recently by large language models. However, routine patient data are often different from other data which is a fact that limits their sheer number. As highly sensitive data are involved, access to personal data, i.e., non-anonymized data, is only permitted either by law or by the patient via informed consent as specified by the EU General Data Protection Regulation [1]. If these data are to be used beyond the original purpose they were captured for, i.e., patient care, permission must be obtained from the patient [1]. Under US law, patient health information is protected by the Health Insurance Portability and Accountability Act (HIPAA) in a corresponding way [2]. Although there are mechanisms such as federated learning to make patient data available for research and AI model training [3], these fundamental restrictions remain in principle. Rare diseases, by their very nature, further limit the data volume that are available [4]. Other problems arise in supervised machine learning when data must be labeled manually by experts because there is no other external source, e.g., histopathology, to objectively validate the ground truth. The time and costs associated with labeling can lead to small datasets if these resources are limited.

Table 13.1 Problems with a small data set

Problem	Definition	Result
Overfitting	Learning from noise and details specific to the data set	Poor performance on new, unseen data
Lack of generalization	Model does not capture the diversity and variability of the underlying data distribution	Less effective in real-world applications
Bias in the data set	Models that might be skewed and discriminatory	Poor performance on new and unseen data
Limited feature representation	Important features or patterns might be missing	Incomplete models
Unreliable evaluation metrics	Standard evaluation metrics, such as accuracy or loss, may not reliably reflect the model's actual performance	Unclear model performance

Given these circumstances, medicine and healthcare—as a domain—seem to be forced to accommodate living with smaller datasets than is usual in machine learning. Small numbers of data records that are used for AI training possess the inherent problem of generalizing the model output poorly [5]. Table 13.1 gives an overview of the problems encountered when using small data sets.

To mitigate the risks due to a small dataset, there are methods that seek to artificially increase the amount of data [6] and comprise, among others, transfer learning, i.e., pre-training the model on large general datasets, such as ImageNet [7] or specialized datasets [8], increasing the number of images through augmentation methods, including synthetic data [9] and cross-validation, increasing the robustness of performance evaluations by splitting the data into multiple training and validation subsets.

In addition to the inherent reasons for small datasets in healthcare, the problems are also due to the fact the data that are spread across departments, institutions, regions, and countries are not interoperable. Interoperability is a critical concept in the context of AI because it directly influences the ability of AI systems to integrate, understand, and utilize diverse data sources and to work within various technological ecosystems. Data integration is achieved through a bundle of interoperability measures ensuring that data from different systems, formats, or standards can be combined seamlessly as shown in the study involving a data integration center from which data for clinical process mining were extracted [10]. The basis of interoperability is the use of common international health IT standards. This embraces the generic health IT standards that are widely used in healthcare such as HL7 FHIR and openEHR as well as terminologies including SNOMED CT.

For more specific use cases, i.e., data sharing for research purposes and AI development, other standards have emerged. Among these standardization initiatives, the Observational Medical Outcomes Partnership (OMOP) has gained much attention in recent years [11]. In general, OMOP aims at standardizing healthcare data to facilitate large-scale observational studies. More specifically speaking, OMOP seeks to create a consistent and standardized way to capture and store healthcare data from diverse sources such as electronic health records (EHRs), insurance

Table 13.2 Simplified OMOP common data model

Standardized clinical data	**Standardized health system**	**Standardized health economics**
Person	Location	Cost
Observational period	Care site	Payer_plan_period
Death	Provider	
Visit occurrences		**Standardized derived data**
Condition occurrences	**Standardized vocabulary**	Condition_era
Drug exposure	Concept	Drug_era
Procedure occurrences	Vocabulary	Dose_era
Device exposure	Domain	**Results schema**
Measurement	Concept_class	Cohort
Observation	Concept_synonym	Cohort_definition
Note	Concept_relationship	
Episode	Relationship	**Standardized metadata**
Specimen	Concept_ancestor	CDM source
Fact relationship	Source_to_concept_map	Metadata
	Drug_strength	

claims, and registries. By standardizing the data format, OMOP enhances interoperability across different healthcare systems and databases, allowing researchers to integrate and analyze data from multiple institutions and data sources.

The key output of OMOP is the OMOP Common Data Model (CDM), which defines a standardized structure for organizing healthcare data (Table 13.2). It enables the transformation of various complex data into a uniform format consisting of tables that capture information about patient conditions, drugs, procedures, measurements, observations, devices, specimens, visits, and the provider. OMOP employs a standardized set of vocabularies for coding and interpreting medical and healthcare data, such as SNOMED CT for clinical terms and LOINC for laboratory tests [12]. Once OMOP CDM compliant data are available from different sources open source tools for data quality and characterization can be applied so that exploratory and hypothesis driven analyses can take place. Enhancing the development of models to predict patient outcomes, disease progression, or treatment responses belongs to the major objectives and use cases of OMOP, and it aligns well with the application areas of AI in healthcare (OMOP CDM) as shown in the literature [13].

In a more general sense, the principles of standardization, interoperability, and a good organization of data are reflected by the concept of FAIR data, whereby FAIR stands for Findable, Accessible, Interoperable, and Reusable [14]. Table 13.3 provides some examples of FAIR data. The FAIRification process (Fig. 13.1) is a centerpiece of research data management and applies to metadata, data, and supporting infrastructures (e.g., search engines) [14].

While measures to ensure findability and accessibility are implemented at the metadata level, interoperability and reuse requirements address the data level. It is an effort that affects stakeholders from various professions and authorities as the example of standardizing data and sharing information about tuberculosis in Brazil to strengthen the national health information systems showed [15].

Table 13.3 Examples of FAIR data applications

FAIR principle	Definition	Example
Findable	Ensuring that healthcare datasets are registered with unique identifiers and indexed in searchable databases enhances their discoverability.	DRYAD repository for open publication and routine reuse of research data [16]
Accessible	Accessibility ensures that crucial health data is available when needed, while still respecting the privacy and security regulations.	Implementations of HIPAA and GDPR rules in organizations
Interoperable	Implementing standardized data formats and healthcare communication protocols.	HL7 FHIR, SNOMED CT
Reusable	Provision of datasets, e.g., under open licenses, with detailed documentation and metadata regarding data collection methods and context.	DRYAD repository for open publication and routine reuse of research data [16] for open data

Data Quality Is First

FAIR data principles are closely linked with the goal to warrant data quality. Improving data quality is a critical task for ensuring that AI developments and data-driven decisions draw on reliable and accurate information. Data quality is defined and expressed by its dimensions including its indicators and metrics [17]:

1. **Accuracy**

   … is defined as the degree to which data correctly describes the "real world" object or event that it represents. It is expressed as structural accuracy, i.e., syntactic wise and semantic wise, and time-related accuracy pertaining to the currency, volatility, and timeliness of the data.

- Metric: The percentage of data entries without errors.

2. **Completeness**

   … is "the extent to which data are of sufficient breadth, depth, and scope for the task at hand" [18]. Completeness refers to relational data (in a database), where values, tuples, attributes, or relations can be missing. It can also refer to other sources of data, e.g., the Web, where completeness has a temporal dimension and is understood as the completability.

- Metric: The ratio of filled data fields versus total fields or the percentage of missing values in a dataset. Completability is measured by how fast the degree of completeness will grow over time.

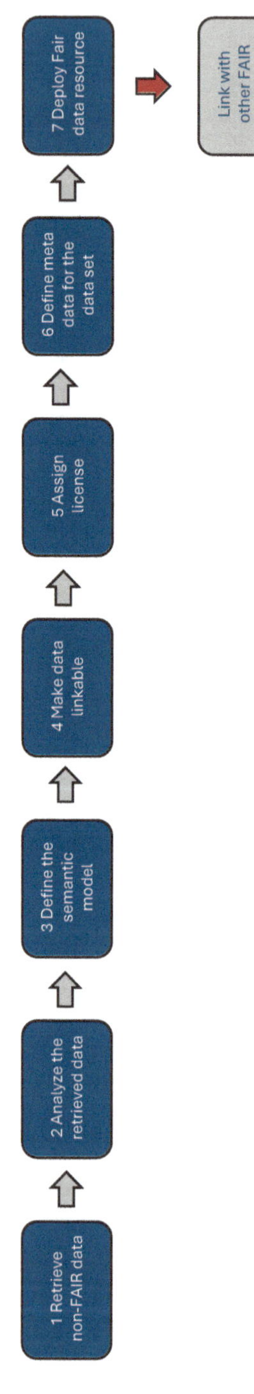

Fig. 13.1 FAIRification process

3. **Accessibility:**
   … is understood as the ease with which data can be obtained and used legally and ethically.
- Metric: The subjective ease of access to data, or the amount of effort and time needed to retrieve data.

4. **Consistency:**
   … is defined as the compliance with semantic rules defined over (a set of) data items, very often it is described as the absence of contradictions within a dataset or among different datasets.
- Metric: The rate of data entries that do not have logical or matched consistency with related data fields or datasets.

Other characteristics as described in Chap. 1 such as

- redundancy including minimality, conciseness, and normalization,
- readability including comprehensibility and clarity,
- usefulness including advantages for the users, and
- trust including reliability and data security [17]

round up the perspective on data quality. It is noteworthy that data quality does not come for free nor is it a pure technical task to guarantee a high level of data quality. Ensuring and improving data quality is a critical task for an organization and its leadership. It heavily relies on data governance policies that are an integral part of this organization. These policies can draw on existing concepts such as the FAIR principles as well as the OMOP common data model and its standardization. They should embrace structural and procedural elements, such as the promotion of a data quality culture, data quality assessment and auditing, comprehensive data documentation, and data quality monitoring, among others.

Data stewards embrace both structural and procedural aspects in their work. Although the role of data stewards is not new, it has gained increasing relevance with the advent of data-driven AI methods and availability of large amounts of data. The responsibilities and duties of data stewards are conceptualized in data governance policies. They embrace data management methods related to the acquisition, storage, aggregation, and de-identification of data and procedures for data provision (procedural elements) [19]. Therefore, some recommendations speak about a FAIR data steward [20].

Conclusions and Outlook

With AI algorithms getting more and more sophisticated, they can be deeply understood only by a few human specialists, and the output sometimes not at all. Conversely, it is the large majority of clinical experts who are producing, collecting, and sometimes labeling the data for training the AI models. They are carrying out quality control together with analytical software and they can perform the plausibility checks of the AI output with critical datasets to challenge these models. It is also human clinical knowledge obtained through data from randomized controlled trials—taking place in the real world—that finds its way into AI models, e.g., large language models, through scientific papers that are used for model training. In other words, human intelligence collectively lays the ground for developing AI applications with data bridging artificial and human intelligence. While we spoke about hardware, software, and peopleware in the past, it is now dataware that we are talking about.

One of the peculiarities of medical and healthcare data is that the data sets can be rather small compared to other domains. There are reasons that are inherent such as data from patients suffering from rare diseases. However, there are also reasons that can be changed, such as the lack of interoperability between information systems and data. Although major advances took place toward greater interoperability, there is still room for improving the technical opportunities to share and reuse data.

Endeavors such as the European Health Data Space (EHDS), the use and exchange of electronic health data across the EU, can serve as a catalyst for data sharing across the entire healthcare spectrum and for data reuse [21]. The EHDS aims at stimulating the primary use of data, i.e., healthcare delivery, including data sharing across borders, and boosting secondary use of data, i.e., the secure and trustworthy reuse of data for research, innovation, and other purposes. This also includes AI developments. Individuals are regarded as the gatekeepers for the access, control, and sharing of their electronic health data. The EHDS is an ambitious undertaking, the implementing of which started in March 2025 when the EHDS Regulation entered into force. Stepwise plans for the implementation of primary use scenarios (2029) and secondary use scenarios (2031) are under way. The EHDS is an example of opening up health data on a very large scale in a trustworthy manner and thereby also offering opportunities for AI systems to be based on truly big data.

In a fundamental sense, data in their dual role as the representatives of the real world and as fuel for AI applications constitute the bridge between the two worlds of artificial intelligence and human intelligence.

Useful Resources

HL7 FHIR. https://www.hl7.org/fhir/

SNOMED CT. https://www.snomed.org/what-is-snomed-ct

Regulation on the European Health Data Space (EHDS). https://ec.europa.eu/newsroom/sante/items/872325/

Reich C, Ostropolets A, Ryan P, Rijnbeek P, Schuemie M, Davydov A, Dymshyts D, Hripcsak G. OHDSI Standardized Vocabularies-a large-scale centralized reference ontology for international data harmonization. J Am Med Inform Assoc. 2024;31(3):583–90. https://doi.org/10.1093/jamia/ocad247.

Wijnbergen D, Kaliyaperumal R, Burger K, Bonino da Silva Santos LO, Mons B, Roos M, Mina E. The FAIR data point populator: collaborative FAIRification and population of FAIR data points. BMC Med Inform Decis Mak. 2025;25(Suppl 1):211. https://doi.org/10.1186/s12911-025-03022-7.

Review Questions

1. What are arguments that speak in favor of data as the link between artificial and human intelligence?
2. What is the meaning of FAIR data and how is it linked with standardization?
3. What are dimensions of data quality?

Answers to Review Questions

1. Data serve in their dual role as the representatives of the real world and as fuel for AI applications and hereby constitute the bridge between the two worlds of artificial intelligence and human intelligence. Data are produced, managed and provided by humans who are responsible for the quality of the data and therefore also for the quality, robustness and validity of the AI output.
2. FAIR stands for Findable, Accessible, Interoperable and Re-usable. It comprises a set of principles and processes for good research data management. Standardization is the key to transforming data into FAIR data and refers to all of the four principles. For example, to make data findable their metadata have to be standardized. Data are accessible in a uniform way if the rules to access the data are applied in a standardized manner. Interoperability relies on the use of (international) communication protocols, health IT standards and standardized terminologies. Re-usability builds on the availability of standardized metadata, interoperable raw data and standardized descriptions of the context of the data.
3. The main dimensions of data quality are accuracy, completeness, accessibility and consistency. Other characteristics such as readability, usefulness, trust and lack of redundancy can be either subsumed by these dimensions or add further perspectives.

References

1. Schütze B. Data protection and data security in the EU: the European general data protection regulation. In: Hübner UH, Wilson GM, Shaw Morawski T, Ball MJ, editors. Nursing informatics: a health informatics, interprofessional and global perspective. Springer; 2022. p. 437–51.
2. Kiel JM. Data privacy and security in the US: HIPAA, HITECH and beyond. In: Hübner UH, Wilson GM, Shaw Morawski T, Ball MJ, editors. Nursing informatics: a health informatics, interprofessional and global perspective. Springer; 2022. p. 427–35.
3. Tang G, Black JE, Williamson TS, Drew SH. Federated diabetes prediction in Canadian adults using real-world cross-province primary care data. AMIA Annu Symp Proc. 2025;2024:1099–108.
4. Omar M, Agbareia R, Naffaa ME, Watad A, Glicksberg BS, Nadkarni GN, Klang E. Applications of artificial intelligence in vasculitides: a systematic review. ACR Open Rheumatol. 2025;7(3):e70016. https://doi.org/10.1002/acr2.70016. PMID: 40091457; PMCID: PMC11911543.
5. Zantvoort K, Nacke B, Görlich D, Hornstein S, Jacobi C, Funk B. Estimation of minimal data sets sizes for machine learning predictions in digital mental health interventions. NPJ Digit Med. 2024;7(1):361. https://doi.org/10.1038/s41746-024-01360-w.

6. Piffer S, Ubaldi L, Tangaro S, Retico A, Talamonti C. Tackling the small data problem in medical image classification with artificial intelligence: a systematic review. Prog Biomed Eng (Bristol). 2024;6(3):ad525b. https://doi.org/10.1088/2516-1091/ad525b.
7. Dührkoop E, Malihi L, Erfurt-Berge C, Heidemann G, Przysucha M, Busch D, Hübner U. Automatic classification of wound images showing healing complications: towards an optimised approach for detecting maceration. Stud Health Technol Inform. 2024;317:347–55. https://doi.org/10.3233/SHTI240877.
8. Hamedi Z, Brigato L, Dack E, Schütz M, Lehmann B, Exadaktylos A, Mougiakakou S, Krummrey G. AI-based analysis of abdominal ultrasound images to support medical diagnosis in emergency departments. Stud Health Technol Inform. 2025;325:16–21. https://doi.org/10.3233/SHTI250209.
9. Abbasi SF, Bilal M, Mukherjee T, Ul Islam S, Pournik O, Arvanitis TN. Preliminary results on improved synthetic image generation for melanoma skin cancer. Stud Health Technol Inform. 2025;323:216–20. https://doi.org/10.3233/SHTI250081.
10. Heidemeyer H, Auhagen L, Majeed RW, Pegoraro M, Bienzeisler J, Peeva V, Beyel H, Röhrig R, van der Aalst WMP, Puladi B. A pipeline for the usage of the core data set of the medical informatics initiative for process mining – a technical case report. Stud Health Technol Inform. 2024;317:30–9. https://doi.org/10.3233/SHTI240835.
11. Observational health data sciences and informatics (OHDSI). Who we are. Available from: https://www.ohdsi.org/who-we-are/. Last access: 26 June 2025.
12. Observational health data sciences and informatics (OHDSI). Standardized data: the OMOP common data model. Available from: https://www.ohdsi.org/data-standardization/. Last access: 26 June 2025.
13. Ahmadi N, Peng Y, Wolfien M, Zoch M, Sedlmayr M. OMOP CDM can facilitate data-driven studies for cancer prediction: a systematic review. Int J Mol Sci. 2022;23(19):11834. https://doi.org/10.3390/ijms231911834.
14. GO FAIR. FAIR principles. Available from: https://www.go-fair.org/fair-principles/. Last access: 26 June 2025.
15. Bernardi F, Lima V, Sartoretto G, Baiochi J, Cassão V, Kritski A, Rijo R, Alves D. From raw data to FAIR data: the FAIRification workflow for Brazilian tuberculosis research. Stud Health Technol Inform. 2023;305:331–4. https://doi.org/10.3233/SHTI230497.
16. DRYAD. Available from: https://datadryad.org/. Last access: 26 June 2025.
17. Batini C, Scannapieco M. Data and information quality – dimensions, principles and techniques. Cham: Springer; 2016. https://doi.org/10.1007/978-3-319-24106-7.
18. Wang RY, Strong DM. Beyond accuracy: what data quality means to data consumers. J Manag Inf Syst. 1996;12(4):5–33. Cited by [17].
19. Rosenbaum S. Data governance and stewardship: designing data stewardship entities and advancing data access. Health Serv Res. 2010;45(5 Pt 2):1442–55. https://doi.org/10.1111/j.1475-6773.2010.01140.x. Epub 2010 Aug 2.
20. de Groot R, van der Graaff F, van der Doelen D, Luijten M, De Meyer R, Alrouh H, van Oers H, Tieskens J, Zijlmans J, Bartels M, Popma A, de Keizer N, Cornet R, Polderman TJC. Implementing findable, accessible, interoperable, reusable (FAIR) principles in child and adolescent mental health research: mixed methods approach. JMIR Ment Health. 2024;11:e59113. https://doi.org/10.2196/59113.
21. European Commission. European Health Data Space (EHDS). Available from: https://health.ec.europa.eu/ehealth-digital-health-and-care/european-health-data-space-regulation-ehds_en. Last access 26 June 2025.

Index

A
Ageing, 110, 111
AI-ageism, 110, 117, 119
AI-enriched care relations, 109, 116–118
AI functional hierarchy, 137
Algorithmic bias, in healthcare AI, 26, 36, 39, 104, 160–162, 166
Artificial intelligence (AI), 4, 9, 10, 19, 26–28, 30, 34, 36, 39, 62, 68, 70, 76, 95–105, 109–119, 132, 136, 147, 157, 164, 165, 170, 171, 174, 180, 183, 186, 190–207, 213, 216, 221, 222
Artificial intelligence (AI) in healthcare, 170, 180, 190–207
Augmentation of human capacities, 4, 20
Automated disease classification, 96, 97, 105
Autonomy, 49, 52, 53, 56, 86, 103, 140, 148, 171, 190, 192, 193, 202, 204–206, 208, 216

B
Barriers and facilitators, 17, 75, 76, 78, 85
Bias, 13–15, 35, 37, 51, 65, 67, 68, 80, 101, 104, 105, 110, 119, 148, 157–166, 172, 175, 177, 181, 185–187, 190, 193, 194, 196, 199, 202, 206, 207, 217
Bias and fairness, 39, 162, 163, 177, 199, 206, 207, 216
Big data, 13, 15, 26, 29, 39, 158, 222
Bioethics, 158
Black box problem in AI, 5, 14, 30, 171, 195, 207

C
Career stages, 61, 63–69, 71, 72
Challenges for AI-assisted decision making, 51, 83
The change process, 61–63, 66, 67, 69, 70, 72
Clinical decision, 82
Clinical decision support, 5, 13, 26, 29, 31
Common morality, 191

D
Data concepts, 142
Data-driven AI, 9, 18, 19, 29–30, 35–36, 185, 221
Data governance, 36, 148, 214, 221
Data quality, 12, 13, 16, 26, 35, 136–138, 143, 164, 185, 214, 219, 221, 223
Data steward, 221
Decision support, 6, 26, 35, 79, 82, 100, 103, 105, 110, 124, 136, 145
Deep learning, 6, 7, 14, 26, 27, 29, 30, 32, 36, 37, 39, 96, 98, 100, 102, 171, 175, 214
Deontology, 191, 192, 202–204
Differential diagnoses, 131
Digitalization, 4, 5, 7, 19
Disembodied AI, 11, 26, 30–31, 38

E
Embodied AI, 11, 26, 30, 31
Emotional intelligence, 44, 47–49, 54, 55, 64, 71, 214
Ethical AI, 26, 27, 34, 36, 38

U. H. Hübner et al. (eds.), *Bridging Artificial and Human Intelligence*, Health Informatics, https://doi.org/10.1007/978-3-032-11938-4

Ethical concerns, 38, 39, 88, 95, 104, 105, 109, 110, 114, 170, 193–197, 200, 202, 204, 216
Ethical guidelines for trustworthy AI, 174, 177, 179, 183
Ethics, 16–18, 148, 177, 179, 180, 183, 191–193, 199, 200, 202–206, 208–209
EU artificial intelligence (AI) act, 164, 170, 174–178, 180, 182, 183, 185–187
Evidence based medicine and nursing, 43, 46, 50
Explainability, 14, 26, 30, 31, 35–37, 39, 53, 102, 148, 171, 174, 180, 183, 208
Explainable AI (XAI), 5, 14, 30, 32, 35, 39, 184, 187, 207

F
FAIR data, 218–223
Future developments, 95, 101, 170

G
General Data Protection Regulation (GDPR), 165, 170, 174, 180, 198, 216
Generative AI, 8, 14, 26, 34, 35, 102, 105, 123–132, 140, 145
Generative pre-trained transformers (GPT), 102, 132
GPT-4, 125, 126, 128, 130–132

H
Health equity, 157–161, 165, 166
Health Insurance Portability and Accountability Act (HIPAA), 165, 179–181, 184, 186, 207, 216, 219
Human decision-making theories, 44–47, 54, 71, 80
Human intelligence, 4, 8–10, 18–20, 28, 43, 44, 47–49, 70, 87, 157, 163, 165, 213–223

I
ICD10 diagnostic codes, 126
Image based diagnostics, 96–97, 105
Implementation outcomes, 79
Implementation research logic model (IRLM), 75, 76, 78–80, 84, 85, 87, 88
Implementation science, 75–88
Informed consent, 36, 39, 81, 104, 171, 185, 186, 190–192, 194, 195, 198, 199, 201, 202, 204, 215, 216
Innovation, 30, 33, 44, 61, 62, 65, 67–70, 78, 98–102, 104, 109, 111, 117, 140, 147, 164, 170, 171, 179, 181–187, 191, 201, 215, 222
Interoperability, 13, 80, 101, 136–138, 141–143, 214, 215, 217, 218, 222

K
Knowledge-based AI, 4, 7–9, 12, 13, 18, 19

L
Large language models (LLMs), 35, 47, 51, 52, 102, 123, 124, 216
Leadership, 61–63, 65, 68–72, 80, 81, 86, 88, 215, 221
Liability for AI in healthcare, 172, 182
Logic models, 75–78, 85, 87, 88

M
Machine learning (ML), 4, 5, 7–9, 11–13, 17–19, 26, 28–33, 38, 39, 83, 84, 97, 98, 100, 111, 113, 124, 139, 140, 145–147, 158, 160, 162, 165, 198, 214, 216, 217
Medical device regulation (MDR), 164, 165, 170, 174, 176, 180
Morality, 191, 202

N
Nursing documentation, 135–150
Nursing workflow, 145

O
Older adults, 109–115, 117–119
OMOP common data model, 142, 214, 218, 221

P
Patient care, 6, 18, 19, 30, 31, 36, 39, 44, 47, 66, 95, 98, 104, 129, 130, 135–150, 170, 173, 176, 193, 195, 197–198, 200–204, 206, 215, 216
Patient–provider relationship, 14, 47–56, 194, 196, 197, 202, 214, 216

Prediction models, 5, 12
Predictive analytics, 29, 31, 38, 83, 98, 104, 105
Principlism
  beneficence, 193
  justice, 193
  non-maleficence, 193

R
Risk mitigation, 82, 135, 136, 140–142, 176
Risks, 4, 12–15, 20, 45, 54, 56, 62, 71, 77, 78, 80, 82, 87, 140, 145, 147, 148, 161, 171, 177, 180, 186, 191, 192, 199, 204–208, 216, 217
Robots, 5, 26, 103, 105, 114, 115, 135, 136, 139, 140, 146, 147, 150
Rule-based AI, 26, 27, 29, 30, 124

S
Skin cancer classification, 105
Small data sets, 217
Social intelligence, 47–49, 55
Statistical methods, 4, 26, 32, 163, 165

T
Tele-dermatology, 96, 98, 104
Thick data, 157, 164–166

U
Utilitarianism, 191, 192, 202–205

V
Virtue ethics, 191, 192, 202–204, 206